Walking Through
the Valley of Dementia

"When you are a care partner for a person living with dementia, finding effective spiritual support is often a challenge. Therese Fisher noticed this and thoughtfully created a tool to help meet this need. For those in the Christian faith, this is an excellent resource for care partners, as well as church communities, chaplains, and other faith-based organizations."

—TEEPA SNOW, founder, Positive Approach to Care®

"Whether you are a care partner for a family member with dementia or a lifelong care partner of dementia patients, ultimate questions of life, its purpose, and its destiny surround you. To find meaning or even to behold God in this work may be a daunting task. Therese Fisher's outstanding book which seamlessly blends current research, personal experience, and sound theological insights offers a self-guided, self-paced retreat for compassionate care partners that strengthens, supports, and nurtures one's spirituality amidst this challenging work."

—GINA HENS-PIAZZA, professor of biblical studies, Jesuit School of Theology of Santa Clara University

"Therese Fisher has brought heaven to earth in this offering. The challenges of being a care partner are often misunderstood, and the options to receive support are few and far between. Bringing her own years of experience as a care partner and understanding of the stresses related to being a carer, Fisher has created a truly usable and easily accessible gift to anyone who seeks respite while walking through the Valley of Dementia."

—ANNE HOUSE, volunteer services manager, Providence Community Health Napa Valley

"This is the kind of book I wish I could have offered to many care partners over the years I worked as a hospice chaplain. Therese Fisher is a compassionate, knowledgeable guide through the terrain of the Valley of Dementia and draws on deep wells of lived experience, advanced study, and Christian wisdom to create much needed retreat for those on a similar path. I know this book will be a beloved companion to many."

—**HEATHER ISAACS**, board certified chaplain

Walking Through the Valley of Dementia

A Self-Paced Spiritual Retreat for Care Partners

THERESE FISHER

RESOURCE *Publications* · Eugene, Oregon

WALKING THROUGH THE VALLEY OF DEMENTIA
A Self-Paced Spiritual Retreat for Care Partners

Resource Publications
An Imprint of Wipf and Stock Publishers
199 W. 8th Ave., Suite 3
Eugene, OR 97401

www.wipfandstock.com

PAPERBACK ISBN: 979-8-3852-1587-4
HARDCOVER ISBN: 979-8-3852-1588-1
EBOOK ISBN: 979-8-3852-1589-8

VERSION NUMBER 05/30/24

For Betsy
Thank you.
I'm sorry.
I forgive you.
I love you.
Bye for now.

Contents

Contents

Contents

Introduction

RATIONALE AND PURPOSE

I HAVE CREATED THIS retreat because I love God. This loving relationship has sustained me as a care partner professionally and personally when society, community, church, and sometimes even family and friends have not been able to. I want to offer other care partners a space where they can explore their relationship with God. I believe that through this relationship, care partners can find nourishment and sustenance for their journey through life in general and specifically through the Valley of Dementia.

God's greatest commandments are to love God with all your heart, soul, and mind and to love your neighbor as yourself (Matt 22:34–40). The generosity that this passage suggests is easy to get lost in, particularly in a care partnering environment. For example, it is "easy" to identify with giving generously to a care partner, to believe we must care for them with every ounce of our being and even that we must suffer for their sake, for the Bible says, "And not only that, but we also boast in our sufferings, knowing that suffering produces endurance, and endurance produces character, and character produces hope." (Rom 5:3–4 NRSVCE) We know God did not promise us an easy road, so we carry on in God's name and forget to care for ourselves.

My firsthand experience and observation of others over the last fifteen years have shown me that the multitude of challenges care partners face often leave them tired and depleted. They (we) don't know where to turn for physical and emotional support, let alone spiritual care, which often falls completely by the wayside. Spirituality and a relationship with God can begin to feel like a luxury that one can abstain from or "put off until after."

The idea of a spiritual retreat might sound refreshing and nourishing. Still, the reality is there often just is not time, or there are no resources available to take an afternoon off, let alone an entire weekend. Studies have shown that successful interventions for caregivers of People Living with Dementia (PLwD) generally have the quality of being individually tailored to them.[1] For that reason, I have compiled this retreat program with various exercises that you, the care partner, can adapt to your own life and use anytime, day or night, at your own pace.

Since most care partners are not professionally trained,[2] my primary focus is on everyday people (family, friends, or acquaintances of the PLwD) who have found themselves in the role of care partner for one reason or another. Though not my primary intended audience, I hope the retreat is also helpful for paid professional care partners.

GOALS

The retreat's primary goal is to nourish and support you, the care partner, through spiritual explorations (such as prayers, meditations, rituals, and journaling) that create a space for you to engage in your relationship with God. Secondary goals include offering some basic education and providing a resource that is easily accessible, low-cost, and self-paced, inviting you to tend to your spirituality in a way that considers your time constraints and other potentially limited resources.

STRUCTURE AND METHODOLOGY

The retreat manual has two main components. The first section lays the groundwork for the retreat, and the second section is the

1. Brodaty and Donkin, "Family Caregivers of People," 222.
2. Brodaty and Donkin, "Family Caregivers of People," 217.

set of retreat exercises. Part one introduces the topic with a vignette of excerpts from the life of a care partner. From there, I provide a basic understanding of dementia and its challenges to help educate and empower care partners. This section is heavily influenced by the "Positive Approach to Care" work founded by Teepa Snow, who has worked in the dementia care field for over four decades.[3] Her methodology combines the science of how the brain works with strategies to care partnering that focus on what the PLwD can do as opposed to what they cannot do. Knowing what is happening in the brain helps us understand a PLwD's reactions and how we can adjust our approaches in ways that promote dignity and positive interactions while reducing stress and aggravation.

Including information about dementia care is integral to the retreat because education has been shown to help improve care partners' mental health and reduce their perceived burden.[4] When an intervention helps a care partner enhance their quality of life, it often also improves the quality of life for the PLwD and delays nursing home placement.[5] In this sense, improving the care partner's quality of life through spirituality can bear the good fruit of Christian social teachings we find in Scripture and from spiritual and other leaders who encourage us to "open [our] hand to the poor and needy" (Deut 15:11) and "support the weak" (Acts 20:35 NRSVCE). We are not isolated beings. We are in a relationship with and dependent on the world around us. Sometimes, a care partner needs support in supporting the life of another.

Part one includes a significant discussion of the challenges of care partnering. This is important for two reasons. The first is to acknowledge the challenge of meeting the care partner where they are and let them know that they are not alone. The second reason to dive into the challenges is that they offer the care partner a profound number of questions about life and about God. In many ways, these questions are the foundation of the retreat. They represent the liminal space traversed in the Valley of Dementia.

3. See www.teepasnow.com.
4. Brodaty and Donkin, "Family Caregivers of People," 223.
5. Brodaty and Donkin, "Family Caregivers of People," 222.

In that way, the questions are more important than the answers in that they are an invitation, an entrance into God's mystery, and into a (deeper) relationship with God.

Part two introduces the retreat format and then the specific retreat exercises. These exercises take the form of journaling, prayers, rituals, and meditations. Prayer and journaling exercises will introduce modified forms of Ignatian prayer, including the Ignatian examen, the colloquy, and imaginative or contemplative prayer, as well as a form of the ancient tradition of Lectio Divina (a style of engaging in scriptural reflection). I do not explicitly name these techniques in the retreat materials because the focus of the retreat is on the care partner engaging in their own spirituality and relationship with the Divine. I name them here to acknowledge how they offer ways of connecting with God and sharing the experience of care partnering with God while inviting God's perspective into the care partner's life. Journaling exercises also allow care partners to engage in their testimony, as modeled by the Psalms. One of the goals behind this is to incorporate the work of Dr. Pennebaker and Dr. Smyth, who argue that sharing one's testimony by means of writing it down can ease stress, reducing the "risk for both major and minor diseases."[6]

In some senses, every part of this retreat is a form of prayer and ritual. Specific written or spoken prayers and practices will allow retreatants to engage in a relationship with God. In his book *Deeply into the Bone*, Ronald Grimes emphasizes the importance of rituals as rites of passage that help us move from who we once were into a new way of being.[7] I hope these rituals will help the retreatant see that the process of care partnering is both a sacred rite of passage in their own personal and spiritual transformation and a sacred act of participation in the PLwD's rite of passage from elder to ancestor.[8]

6. Pennebaker and Smyth, *Opening Up*, 1.

7. Grimes, *Deeply into the Bone*, 7.

8. "Elderhood is such a series of losses. It would [be amazing if we] knew how to ritualize and honor people in this liminal space between elder and ancestor . . . so that they can leave their body one offering at a time." Fleurdujon, "Rite of Passage."

PART ONE

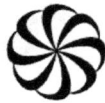

The Valley of Dementia

1

Terminology

IN THIS RETREAT, I use the abbreviation "PLwD" for Person or People Living with Dementia. I was introduced to this phrase by Teepa Snow, a leader in the field of dementia care, who recommends using it over terms like "dementia patient," which emphasize the symptom and not the person. I use it here because it aligns with my value of person-centered care. As Snow points out, "Dementia isn't what defines a person and it isn't a choice. Instead, it is a condition that the person, and those around them, are learning to live with and constantly adapt to."[1] It is not my intention to reduce people to a set of letters. Each person living with dementia is a unique child of God. I use the abbreviation simply to minimize the number of times the phrase "Person Living with Dementia" is written out.

Also, in this retreat, I will use the term "care partner" instead of "caregiver" unless directly quoting or referencing a study that identifies its participants using the term "caregiver." When I refer to a care partner, I refer to the subset of care partners caring for PLwD, as that is the focus for this retreat. The reasons for using the term "care partner" instead of "caregiver" are twofold. First, although the term "caregiver" is undoubtedly more commonly used today, it connotes one person doing something for or to another.

---

1. Snow, *Understanding the Changing Brain*, xii.

The term "care partner" emphasizes that relationality should be our primary focus. Snow suggests a shift in philosophy from "doing for and to" to a philosophy of "helping with and partnering with"[2] helps to create a more positive experience for all involved.

The second reason I use the term "care partner" is because its focus on relationships aligns more with Christian social teaching. In *Evangelii Gaudium*, Pope Francis called for all Christians to be disciples and missionaries. "Being a disciple means being constantly ready to bring the love of Jesus to others, and this can happen unexpectedly and in any place . . . [this] is always respectful and gentle, the first step is personal dialogue when the other person speaks and shares his or her joys, hopes and concerns for loved ones, or so many other heartfelt needs."[3] The term "care partner" mimics Pope Francis' message of being in personal dialogue with someone, and the journey of dementia is full of unexpected moments and opportunities for those dialogues (that may or may not happen with words). Pope Francis says, "We should not think, however, that the Gospel message must always be communicated by fixed formulations learned by heart or by specific words which express an absolutely invariable content."[4] His words here echo the idea of not doing "for" or "to" someone, not deciding what they need without their input, but instead sharing with them and learning to collaborate in a journey of partnership. In this way, I believe care partners are able to bring the gospel message alive in unique ways.

Lastly, I want to acknowledge my terminology around the name of God. I have made every effort to separate gender from God's identity. Whether gender is "ultimate truth" or a social construct, I will not take the time to explore here. I do believe that nothing can separate us from the love of God, including gender or gender identity, and that God is something more vast than a gender category. As clumsy and cumbersome as it can be to discuss God, God's will, and God's teaching without pronouns, I don't want a patriarchal imagination to alienate retreat participants or

2. Snow, *Understanding the Changing Brain*, xi.

3. Pope Francis, *Evangelii Gaudium*, §127–28.

4. Pope Francis, *Evangelii Gaudium*, §129.

diminish the vastness of God's mystery and how or through whom God might communicate with them. I have also tried to remove names such as "Lord," "Master," or "Savior" unless in a direct quote. I have a deep appreciation for these faces of God, and I am uncomfortable using these particular names here as they can trap me (and others) in the pain of submission and violation caused by human beings and human systems. If these names of God liberate and inspire you, please take space to write them and use them in your retreat. If the names I use trigger you, try other designations based on where you find vast sacredness and expansive love throughout your retreat journey. Maybe even use your own secret nickname for the Big Holy.

2

Vignette

WHILE ON A TRIP, a daughter got up early to find her mom sitting on the kitchen floor surrounded by pots, pans, and other kitchen accouterments. Mom had pulled everything out of the cabinets and was rummaging through them. When the daughter asked what she was doing, the mom looked around at the mess. Then, she suddenly announced that she likes to leave a place cleaner than she found it, and since she could not sleep, she might as well reorganize the kitchen.

Two women at a restaurant walked together to the restroom. One of the two went into the stall and used the toilet but then wouldn't come out. She would not leave the stall. She would not and could not unlock the door. The other woman stood there in the bathroom, horrified, praying, and fighting back tears. "God, help us. Please help her to remember how to open the door. I can't lift it. I can't force the door. I don't want to go out and get help and have everyone know that I can't take care of her anymore, that she can't take care of herself. Help her not to be afraid and panic like I am right now." After a very long time the woman somehow unlocked and left the stall. Exhausted and disoriented, they left the restroom and were surprised to be greeted by her pastor and his son. Smiles. Everything is fine.

A care partner takes a woman out shopping at one of her favorite stores. The woman picks out some things to try on, and they go into the dressing room together. The woman takes off her clothes and then becomes confused and will neither try on the clothing she brought in nor put her original clothing back on. The care partner cannot leave this woman alone and so cannot go out for help. And what could she say if someone walked by? She could not invite a stranger into the dressing room and violate this half-naked woman's privacy and dignity. She slides down to the floor, helpless and hopeless, and prays for divine intervention.

A care partner goes to check on someone only to discover they are not there. They have wandered off. There is a sense of complete and utter panic; anything could have happened. There is a deep feeling of failure; it is all the care partner's fault, "if only I had [fill in the blank]." The family is gathered, and search parties head out.

The care partner in these stories is me, and the woman I am sharing this journey with is my stepmother, Betsy. She started showing signs of dementia around twelve years ago. She was diagnosed with Alzheimer's disease a few years after that. As I write this, Betsy is bedridden with Alzheimer's and has been on hospice for over a year. She has aphasia (difficulty understanding or using words) and so hasn't been able to use language effectively for more than five years. For years after that scene in the restaurant, I would pause each time I saw my pastor's son and would be instantly transported back in that bathroom and feel the horror, panic, and shame wash over me again. Now, when I see him, a different feeling washes over me. I smile and long for those days when Betsy could use words. I hunger for the days when she knew who I was. I'm even beginning to feel a deep sense of gratitude arise in me that at some point in the vastness of time, this woman knew my name, that she chose me to be a part of her family, and that I got to love her and be loved by her.

I thought that I was prepared for this journey. I have worked in hospice for more than fifteen years. I have been trained as a certified nursing assistant (CNA). I am a person-centered care specialist for an Adult Day Health program, which provides care for adults suffering from acute or chronic illness and/or dementia.[1] I

1. "Adult Day Health," lines 1–2.

have seen and experienced so much related to dementia. I thought I would have a sense of solid ground. Still, this journey has been excruciating for me. Though there are resources to help with care techniques, social/emotional support, and encouragement for "self-care," I have found few dementia-specific resources readily available for the spiritual support of care partners. So I offer you what I could not find in the hopes that your steps might be more graceful than mine and so that you find yourself in a deeper relationship to the ultimate source of love and nourishment.

3

What is Dementia?

DEMENTIA IS OFTEN MISUNDERSTOOD and not talked about openly. Yet, the World Health Organization (WHO) says, "More than 55 million people have dementia worldwide, over 60% of whom live in low-and middle-income countries."[1] As we start to explore what dementia is, let's begin by looking at what dementia is not. First, as we advance in age, like many other parts of our body, our brain often does not respond as quickly or work quite as well as it did when we were younger. This is not dementia; it is normal aging.

Second, dementia is not a disease or a diagnosis. Generally, the signs of dementia appear, and then doctors try to diagnose the cause of those signs and symptoms. There are over 120 types, forms, or causes of dementia,[2] including Alzheimer's disease, Lewy body dementia, Parkinson's disease, vascular dementia, genetic predisposition, and brain injury, each with its indicators and symptoms.

Third, dementia isn't one specific symptom. Dementia is a type of brain change, and our brains are complex systems. The part of the brain that is changing will influence how a person's body manifests the symptoms unique to them. General patterns can unfold, but it is essential to remember that each person's expression

---

1. "Dementia," line 1.
2. Snow, *Understanding the Changing Brain*, xii.

9

of dementia is unique to them. In addition, the rate at which the changes occur varies from person to person. This makes the job of care partnering a very dynamic and demanding experience.

So now that we have an idea of what dementia is not, let's talk about what dementia is and what it looks like. Dementia is a type of brain change. In part because of fears around dementia, many people have forgotten that brain changes are normal. Our brains don't work as efficiently when we are tired or hungry. We might get irritable or become unable to focus. When a car cuts us off on the freeway, when we hear a piercing alarm, or when we begin to feel an earthquake, the chemistry in our brain changes and causes us to react in different ways. These brain changes are a normal part of life's rhythm. The difference between these kinds of brain changes and dementia is that a healthy brain returns to normal functioning given sufficient recovery time. The brain of a PLwD does not have the capacity for that recovery. They are experiencing *neurodegeneration.*[3]

This doesn't mean that every time the brain changes its state, a PLwD experiences permanent decline; for example, the brain doesn't function the same when we are asleep versus awake. This is a normal rhythm of change. But when there is a decline in a PLwD, neither their brain nor current medical science has a methodology for regaining that function. Snow describes the difference between a "healthy brain" and one with dementia as a difference in elasticity.[4] A brain with dementia does not have the elasticity that a normal functioning brain has.

Dr. Ayati, a gerontologist and medical advisor to the United States Senate Special Committee on Aging, uses a bank analogy.[5] The brain has limited functioning units (neurons) deposited in its bank. When you run out of money in your bank account, you don't typically run to the mall or go on a shopping spree. You conserve your funds and slowly withdraw them only to pay for the

3. The neurons in the brain are deteriorating and dying. Snow, *Understanding the Changing Brain*, 7.

4. Snow, *Understanding the Changing Brain*, xv.

5. Ayati, in conversation with author, May 19, 2023.

necessities (food, rent, utilities). So, too, as the brain runs out of neurons, it stops "spending" its resources on non-essential functions so that it can keep the heart and lungs working.

At first, the effects of this might not be noticeable, like mixed-up words or using poor judgment, something anyone might do. The effects become more apparent and potentially harmful as things progress. According to Snow, the early signs of dementia are the following:

- The person can't always restrain the desire to say or do what they would like rather than what is socially expected of them.

- The person does not get the message being sent in the words or phrases being used due to inaccurate or inadequate connections between semantic memories and the current event.

- The person can no longer reason through a complex social situation or unfamiliar environment and so makes errors in behavior based on a partial understanding or faulty cause-and-effect reasoning.

- The person loses the ability to look at a situation from multiple viewpoints as well as the ability to take familiar information, reorganize it, and categorize it in a new or unusual way.[6]

These changes can become more pronounced as the brain continues its decline, and it can become difficult to manage money, pay bills, or keep a regular sleep schedule. One can find oneself wandering or getting lost as one becomes less able to recognize people, places, and/or things. As the decline progresses, symptoms might be loss of balance, lost or reduced senses (taste, touch, smell, hearing, vision), an inability to walk, incontinence, or the loss of language ability (aphasia). In the end stages, the body doesn't have enough neurons for things such as wound healing or swallowing functions.[7] To look at this from a care partner's perspective, what

---

6. Snow, *Understanding the Changing Brain*, 22.

7. It is important to remember here that different dementias will see declines in different parts of the brain and so symptoms will not be the same for everyone. For example, some people with dementia can still function as a

this means is that there is not one list of "job duties" that applies throughout the entire dementia journey because every day, every moment, the brain of the PLwD is shifting and changing, and the care partner must constantly adapt.

To move from the more general definition of dementia being a type of brain change and how we might experience that to something more of a clinical definition, the umbrella term of dementia means four things (regardless of the type of dementia).[8] First, there are at least two parts of the brain that are dying. This means that "the person's ability to successfully [and I will add safely] interpret the environment and select and perform the socially acceptable [and safe] role is gradually lost."[9] Second, there is progression. Things continue to change for the worse. Third, dementia is chronic; that is to say, there is no cure, at least at this point. And fourth, dementia is terminal; the end result is death. In fact, according to the WHO, it is "the seventh leading cause of death and one of the major causes of disability and dependency among older people globally."[10]

---

high-powered lawyer but are unable to put a shirt on a clothes hanger. Some will have delusions, some will not. Some will change their personality, some will not.

8. Snow, *Understanding the Changing Brain*, 17.

9. Snow, *Understanding the Changing Brain*, 19.

10. "Dementia," line 5.

4

Care Partners and Their Challenges

IN THIS SECTION, I will focus on who care partners are and what kinds of challenges they experience. From my perspective as a care partner, professionally and personally, I have seen four primary areas where care partners can become depleted: financially, physically, mentally/emotionally, and spiritually. The first three will be addressed in this chapter, and the last, spirituality, will be discussed in chapter 5. Though I break the discussion into different chapters, these challenges are interconnected; the experience of a deficiency in one can exacerbate any of the others, and many life factors can complicate them.

Before going on, I want to acknowledge that I am a white, cisgender, heterosexual woman in a middle-income household in the United States of America who was raised Catholic and is an active member of multiple Christian congregations (primarily Baptist and Catholic). Because of my situation in life, I have rights, privileges, and biases that I am not always aware of. I speak from my own experiences with the aid of research as I discuss these challenges and acknowledge that I cannot and would not try to speak for everyone's experience. I have been working in a traditionally underpaid and undervalued profession, mainly comprised of women of color. There are many implications of care partnering relating to race, ethnicity, sexuality, and socioeconomic status that, while incredibly important, I cannot adequately address in this retreat.

If you are caring for a PLwD, you, too, are living with dementia. You might not live with it inside your body but are engaged in an active relationship with it. It is a significant part of your life. You may have chosen this role, found yourself in it unexpectedly, or even felt that it was forced upon you. You might see the work of care partnering as a form of ministry, a calling from God, a profound honor, a gift for a loved one, a duty, a source of income, a heavy and unwanted burden, or quite likely some combination of these or other factors. Regardless of how dementia has come into your life, your relationship with it is changing who you are. And change brings with it both gifts and challenges. A 2005 study of caregivers of people living with Alzheimer's reported that 81 percent of caregivers described having both challenges and receiving gifts, or as they refer to it in the study, "gains." Some of those "gains" included personal growth, enjoying togetherness and sharing, feeling a reciprocal bond, feelings of accomplishment and mastery, and spiritual growth.[1] Though this retreat will focus on spirituality, I hope that in doing so, you can see and connect with some of these other gifts more readily.

FINANCIAL CHALLENGES

Approximately 75 percent of caregiving is done informally by family members or friends,[2] who, according to the World Health Organization, provide an average of five hours of care and supervision daily.[3] In the United States, 60 percent of caregivers also have other jobs.[4] Since dementia is progressive, the PLwD has increased care needs as time passes.[5] This can negatively affect a care partner's finances by reducing income, increasing expenses,

1. Sanders, "Is the Glass Half Empty," 57–73.
2. Brodaty and Donkin, "Family Caregivers," 217.
3. "Dementia," line 6.
4. Brodaty and Donkin, "Family Caregivers," 220.
5. According to the Alzheimer's Society, people live on average between six and ten years, depending on the type of dementia. See "Later Stage of Dementia."

or both. Reduced earnings happen when care partners must leave a job, reduce hours, or even turn down promotions at their paying jobs to be with the PLwD. Increased expenses, assuming one has at least some insurance coverage, can range from increased gas bills and vehicle maintenance (from additional driving between households or on errands) to increased grocery bills to needing to pay for adaptive clothing, medical equipment, or other outside services (for either themselves or the PLwD) not covered by insurance or Medicare.

PHYSICAL CHALLENGES

From a physical perspective, a care partner's body can become tired from the hard physical work of assisting with activities of daily living (ADLs), such as transferring, bathing, walking, dressing, cooking, cleaning, feeding, and toileting. Since most care partners for PLwD are not trained professionals, they likely have other jobs or regular responsibilities such as parenting, and the combination of these activities can be physically draining. Lack of training can also mean being more injury-prone while assisting PLwD with ADLs. It is no wonder that care partners have significantly lower health-related quality of life.[6] Care partners of PLwD have an increased risk of various health problems such as cardiovascular problems, reduced immune function, and slower wound healing, and "report a greater number of physical health problems and worse overall health compared with noncaregiver controls."[7] Since women provide 70 percent of total care hours,[8] women's health is disproportionally affected.[9]

6. Shin and Kim, "Family Caregivers," 1.

7. Brodaty and Donkin, "Family Caregivers," 220.

8. "Dementia," lines 7–8.

9. Note that some studies show the percentage of male caregivers is increasing. Brodaty and Donkin, "Family Caregivers," 217–18.

PSYCHOLOGICAL/EMOTIONAL CHALLENGES

From a psychological/emotional perspective, the mind can become tired from constantly watching for safety concerns or signs of change. Care partners are continually reevaluating what is needed, how much autonomy the PLwD desires and can reasonably manage, thinking of new ways to approach situations, and trying to balance between lessons learned from past interactions versus allowing what is happening now to be its own unique experience and approaching it with fresh eyes.

Additional stressors to mental well-being can come from juggling multiple demands of work, family, church, hobbies, a social life, and community obligations and from things such as quality of relationship with the care partner, other stressful life events happening simultaneously, the care partner's physical and mental health, overall life satisfaction, and self-esteem.[10] These kinds of experiences (worries, uncertainties, and overwhelm) might be why several studies have shown a correlation between caring for PLwD and depression and anxiety (between 23 percent and 85 percent experience depression, and between 16 percent and 45 percent experience anxiety.)[11]

Emotional exhaustion for care partners can also manifest as and derive from social isolation and grief. Just as the brain begins to shut down with the progression of dementia, our life's system of organization begins to shut down. We eliminate things we don't feel necessary for survival, like time spent with friends, attending church, or community involvement. Other times, social isolation might not be a time management issue, but deliberately avoiding people out of shame or embarrassment surrounding dementia or out of a sense of inadequacy. Conversely, friends, family, and community members might avoid the care partner because of embarrassment, discomfort, or other life factors.

10. Brodaty and Donkin, "Family Caregivers," 219.
11. Brodaty and Donkin, "Family Caregivers," 219.

Psychiatrist Bessel van der Kolk describes trauma as "when we are not seen and known."[12] This means that social isolation deriving from care partnering can indeed be traumatizing. Gabor Maté, author of *The Myth of Normal: Trauma, Illness and Healing in a Toxic Culture*, argues that "Trauma Fosters a Shame-Based View of the Self."[13] If this is true and shame leads to social isolation and social isolation is a form of trauma by not being seen and known, then social isolation becomes a negative cycle spiraling into darkness.

Feelings of grief can arise from seeing people in a constant and ever-changing state of decline and from the experience of losing the PLwD a little more each day. As the care partner confronts mortality, it can lead to a reassessment of values and beliefs, which sometimes means letting go of things we hold dear.

Something can happen to a care partner as they witness someone else's pain, suffering, and decline. Over time, this can build up and is called "compassion fatigue" or "vicarious trauma."[14] Another trauma-related complication that often happens when we are stretched too thin is that we begin to loosen our hold on pain, trauma, or discomfort from the past. When the resources that we once used to keep these things in check, at bay, or repressed get reassigned to caregiving duties, we might experience unresolved grief, pain, or trauma. As these feelings pop up, in our diminished state, it can feel like we are in a room of one thousand kittens, all crying to be fed simultaneously.

ADDITIONAL COMPLICATIONS

As we have seen, complications can stem from within our lives. Some also are from the outside and larger social structures. On the individual level, the average five hours of care provided each day, as mentioned previously, can mean less sleep, less time for

12. Maté and Maté, *Myth of Normal*, loc. 530.
13. Maté and Maté, *Myth of Normal*, loc. 632.
14. Day and Anderson, "Compassion Fatigue," 1.

emotional support, less time for social connectedness, and/or less time for exercise. In the realm of things outside our control that add complications, there are earthquakes, fires, pandemics, or other unexpected tragedies. On the social structure level, there are complications relating to the systems we find ourselves living in. Dementia is more prevalent in low- and middle-income countries, and low and middle-income families are less likely to be able to afford paid care partners or assisted living facilities. Additionally, cultural values and traditions can make it harder for a particular individual to have positive care partnering experiences.

One major social structure that impacts dementia care is racism in the United States. "Socially entrenched bigotry, whether in its subtle or overt forms, takes an enormous and, until very recently, mostly unspoken toll on health."[15] This can mean, for example, that people of color do not receive the same level of physical care and emotional support as their white counterparts. As true as this is for the PLwD, it is also true for their care partner. Care partners might not receive the same level of respect or support services in their role because of the systemic and personal biases of those offering that support.

15. Maté and Maté, *Myth of Normal*, loc. 4851.

5

Spiritual Challenges in the Valley of Dementia

THE FINAL CATEGORY OF challenges I want to address is spirituality. On an average day, most of us have difficulties in our spiritual life. Our relationship with God grows and changes, our understandings evolve, we discover new, seemingly unanswerable questions, and we struggle with forgiveness, acceptance, and loving one another. In the Valley of Dementia, these experiences can amplify, if not grow exponentially.

One could easily make a case that the spiritual challenges associated with care partnering are all based on emotion. To understand them more clearly, I will break them into smaller categories: physical, emotional, intellectual, and relationship with God. Each of these categories will interrelate and intertwine just as the challenges in the previous section do. I am using the physical class to refer to spiritual challenges that pertain to our physical being in the world. Emotional spiritual challenges are the common emotional reactions we have to care partnering PLwD that relate to our sense of personhood and spirituality. Intellectual spiritual challenges arise from the discord between whom we think we should be, whom our faith or our church/religion says we should be, and the reality of our situation. The last category, relationship with God, often spills over from the intellectual challenges but pertains specifically to our personal relationship with God. Because the care relationship with the PLwD is a partnership, the lines can be blurred between what one witnesses and what one experiences. What the care partner sees and experiences and how they interpret these things can complicate the challenges.

SPIRITUAL CHALLENGES: PHYSICAL

Many physical changes occur when dementia enters the life of a care partner. As discussed earlier, there can be a loss of or distancing from the church or one's spiritual community. Separation can stem from inner changes, such as feelings of shame, embarrassment, or insufficiency. It might also come from outside circumstances. You might not have time to attend church or community events with all the care duties. Church attendance might not be possible because the PLwD can no longer conform to the social norms of the ritual itself. They might get up and wander or speak out at inappropriate times. Pastor Robert Davis shares some of the issues he ran into in his congregation while ministering to PLwD. The PLwD can become agitated or angry as they lose the ability to see, hear, and understand the liturgy, so things that once were comforting are now signs of something being wrong or broken. The PLwD might become aggressive and angry at something a parishioner or the pastor/priest says. They might shift their beliefs or believe you have brought them to the wrong church.[1]

All of these things can accumulate in the physical loss of community and community support. But it is more significant than just the loss of community; it is physical separation from full participation in the liturgy. John F. Baldovin, S.J., offers ten reasons why we go to mass:

1. participation in the world's salvation,

2. the experience of the Glory of God—the experience of humans fully alive in Christ,

1. Davis and Davis, My Journey, 17.

3. learning/practicing discipline of faith,

4. hearing the Scriptures communally,

5. developing a moral life, where we learn how to mirror the generosity and love of Christ,

6. companionship with Christ,

7. focusing on our needs by placing them individually and communally on the altar,

8. praying for the world, where we can look beyond our circumstances and pray for God's creation,

9. welcoming the kingdom of God, where we invite and celebrate our being made new in the arrival of God's reign and salvation, and

10. the experience of joy as we receive Jesus through the eucharist.[2]

I am not saying that one cannot experience some of these outside the formal mass. Still, if we expect and believe that mass "is the summit toward which the activity of the Church is directed; at the same time, it is the font from which all her power flows,"[3] then our loss of church community feels like a physical separation from God, God's feast, God's peace, God's blessing, God's people, and God's salvation of the world.

SPIRITUAL CHALLENGES: EMOTIONAL

The emotional challenges of care partnering relate to our sense of personhood and spirituality. Here, we begin to see a twofold nature to the care partners' challenges. There are challenges that we feel pressing in on our lives from earthly burdens, and there are invitational challenges where God bids us enter into a new way of being. One can feel inadequate as a care partner or a human being and simultaneously have the complementary challenge of trust in God.

---

2. Baldovin, *Bread of Life*, 189–92.

3. Paul VI, "Sacrosanctum Concilium," §10.

As a care partner, you have a front-row seat to someone's process of changing or disintegrating selfhood. Neurological science's concept of mirror neurons might be helpful here. Mirror neurons are a "class of neurons that discharge both when an individual executes a motor act and when he observes another individual performing the same or a similar motor act."[4] Care partners can use this phenomenon to trigger an action from a PLwD when that person doesn't consciously remember how to do it.[5] Additionally, intentionally mirroring a person's concern or worry can help them feel safe and understood. Snow calls this, taking their side by matching their level of distress.[6] However, mirror neurons are not something that we necessarily consciously control. So, when a care partner sees the decline or distress in the PLwD, consider what might be happening with their mirror neurons and how that might invite them to explore their own death and decline (either the physical body or the end of some aspect of life). In a sense, our mirror neurons are inviting us to explore a range of emotions and spiritual challenges we wouldn't otherwise be engaging in.

Some of the challenging things care partners see are that the PLwD loses their dignity, identity, and ability to express desires and needs. You might witness their infantilization (being treated as an infant instead of an adult), their feelings of failure, anxiety, anger, worthlessness, confusion, or paranoia. You might watch them become "useless" when whatever they identify as their spiritual gifts or as their contribution to society vanishes. In all this, the care partner can confront their mortality. At the same time, God asks us to see God's beauty unfold in new and unexpected ways. God invites us to see our care partner new each day. We are faced with letting go of who the PLwD was, asked not to dwell on the past, and invited to watch God make something new (Isa 43:18–19). There is the challenge that God is slowly taking them away from us *and* the invitation to remember that God is also drawing them ever closer.

4. Acharya and Shukla, "Mirror Neurons," 118–24.

5. Shapiro, "Mirroring Care."

6. Feurich, "10 Steps to De-Escalating."

Pastor Davis gives us unique insight into the emotional challenges of a PLwD in his book *My Journey into Alzheimer's Disease*. He describes feelings that he and others he ministered to have gone through on their Alzheimer's journey: God doesn't love them anymore, God is punishing them, and that is why they have Alzheimer's; they are no longer worthy of God's love, and so, there is a fear of death because they must no longer be welcome in God's kingdom. On top of all that, there is the emotional stress and guilt caused by being the focus of well-meaning loved ones "who sincerely feel that by their spiritual exhortations they can force Christ to penetrate into their loved one's troubled mind"[7] or who sincerely want to help, but don't know how (the PLwD becomes a symbol and a source of their hopelessness).

As his life with Alzheimer's progressed, he describes the devastation of being unable to "pray as I wanted because my emotions were dead and cut off."[8] He shares:

> Now I discovered the cruelest blow of all. This personal and tender relationship that I had with the Lord was no longer there. This time of love and worship was removed. There were no longer any feelings of peace and joy. I cried out to God for it to be restored. I howled out to the Lord to come back and speak to my spirit as he had done before. This was unfair and unthinkable. I could only cry out bitterly to the Lord, "Why God, why? How can you leave me at a time like this? Is there some unpardonable sin that I have unconsciously committed? O God, I have lost so much already! How can you take this last joy from me?"[9]

The mirroring, the witnessing, and the experiencing of the PLwD's decline can inspire stages of grief that can manifest spiritually: denial, anger, bargaining, depression, acceptance, and finding meaning.[10] We can be angry at God for what God is putting us through and the PLwD. We can silence God or deny that God is

7. Davis and Davis, *My Journey*, 108.
8. Davis and Davis, *My Journey*, 53.
9. Davis and Davis, *My Journey*, 47.
10. David Kessler, *Finding Meaning*.

any part of our lives. We can bargain with God (if only God would heal the PLwD), and we can become depressed about feeling a lack of God's presence in our lives. With God's help, we can also accept what is going on. We can even find graces and meaning along the journey through the Valley of Dementia. Engaging in an intimate relationship with God that includes honesty and openness about our feelings can help.

SPIRITUAL CHALLENGES: INTELLECTUAL

Throughout the history of Christianity, people have been experiencing Christ and writing about it in the hopes that others can share in that experience, too. They tell us to speak the name of Jesus, read/memorize scripture, or pray a certain way. Most of these teachings have come through those with a highly functional intellectual ability. They make good sense when one's cognitive skills are robust. When cognition is declining however, these same teachings and advice can seem insulting, exclusionary, or, at the very least, raise a lot of (ironically) intellectual challenges. One can begin to ask deep questions that challenge the nature of our lives, our values, and what it means to be a good Christian because, as care partners, we share the journey and the big questions of the PLwD while also asking our own.

A care partner might ask, "If the PLwD can no longer do all of the things a 'good' Christian should do, are they no longer a 'good' Christian? If they are still a 'good' Christian, and they aren't doing those things, then how can my doing them mean that I am a 'good' Christian? If I have known God through myself and my understanding, what happens when that goes away? Do I no longer know God? Does God no longer know or love me?" This section explores the questions that constitute our spiritual challenges to God and God's invitations to us.

The book of Romans asserts, "If you confess with your lips that Jesus is Lord and believe in your heart that God raised him from the dead, you will be saved" (Rom 10:8–9 NRSVCE). When one experiences aphasia, the loss of the ability to use or understand words, how can one meet this criteria of being in a relationship with God and being "saved"? How can one believe in Jesus when one does not have the cognitive ability to understand what belief is or the memory to know who Jesus is? It seems God offers us a different challenge: to trust what cannot be known, that there are more ways for belief and confession to unfold than what we readily see and understand.

The Pontifical Biblical Commission's document "What is Man?" tells us, "Interpretation [of the Bible] is, or rather must be, an act of obedience."[11] Suppose the portions of the brain that maintain the ability to obey or interpret have died. How might this edict be followed? To interpret the Bible requires reading the Bible or listening to it. As dementia advances, these things can become impossible, as can remembering memorized scriptures. Here, I believe, God invites us into vast mystery. Can we enter where God beckons us, to that place where we have enough, where weakness is not darkness, where "my grace is sufficient for you, for my power is made perfect in weakness" (2 Cor 12:9 NIV)? Can we learn to engage in a relationship with God using different methods and senses so that when our abilities shift, our relationships are not cut off but renewed?

"Pray without ceasing" (1 Thess 5:17 NAB), Scripture tells us. That is the right way to pray. Theologian Dietrich Bonhoeffer says, "When our will wholeheartedly enters into the prayer of Christ, then we pray correctly. Only in Jesus Christ are we able to pray. And with him, we also know that we shall be heard. And so we must learn to pray."[12] How can one *not* feel hopeless when they can no longer learn, remember how, or know how to pray? Are they no longer "in [God's] image, according to [God's] likeness" (Gen 1:26 NAB)? Christians are taught constantly to pray the words of Jesus to God "not my will but yours be done" (Luke 22:42b NAB). What happens when the brain declines to the point of being unable to control impulses and desires or to feel emotions as one did in past experiences of God?

11. Pontifical Biblical Commission, "What Is Man?," §5.
12. Bonhoeffer and Brueggemann, *Psalms*, 02:42.

As we struggle with these questions, can we also accept God's invitation to trust that we are made in God's image, even in our brokenness, decline, and dying? Can we allow it to be true when God says, "I will put my laws in their minds, and I will write them upon their hearts" (Heb 8:10b NAB)? Can we trust that God has put what we need inside us even when we do not know how to access or use it? According to Jesus, God's greatest commandment is "You shall love the Lord, your God, with all your heart, with all your soul, and with all your mind" (Matt 22:37 NAB). God doesn't specify an IQ or a level of cognitive or physical functionality; we just love God with everything we have. Can we trust that whatever remains in us and in our PLwD is enough? Can we trust that our coming together in caring partnership is honoring God's command to love one another (John 15:17)? And if so, can we allow ourselves to receive the promise that God is there in the midst of us (Matt 18:20)?

CHALLENGES IN OUR RELATIONSHIP WITH GOD

For many Christians, we dearly cherish our relationship with God. We want to be like the angels who seem to have the favor of God, who prostrate themselves and declare, "Amen. Blessing and glory, wisdom and thanksgiving, honor, power, and might be to our God forever and ever. Amen" (Rev 7:12 NAB). We think this is how we must be to be in "right relationship" with God; it must be a personal relationship, or the relationship has to look a certain way. We strive and yearn for this. Ultimately, the questions seem to come down to what it means to be worthy of God's love and how we maintain a relationship with God when we don't know how to be in a relationship.

We build our relationships based on common experiences, shared beliefs, and characteristics we like. Maybe we enjoy someone's smile, sense of humor, how they make us feel, the nice things they do for us, or how they stand up for us and help us when we are in need. What is the relationship based on if those things disappear? A PLwD can forget who their spouse is or who their children are, and they can certainly lose the ability to display the characteristics we love. So, too, they can forget who Jesus or God is, and then what? It is easy for the care partner and the PLwD to feel abandoned by God.

Is God inviting us to question our fundamental assumptions about what it means to love someone and instead ask what love God calls us to in this moment? Can we trust that nothing can separate us from the love of God (Rom 8:38–39)? Can we embrace a new kind of unconditional love that doesn't require someone to be in a healthy, recognizable body or even in a body at all?

Perhaps you are feeling overwhelmed with questions and challenges at this point. I have presented you with a lot; you probably have more of your own. If so, take a deep breath. You are not alone. Remember that the questions are doorways to finding God. As the poet Rilke says, "Try to love the questions themselves, like locked rooms and like books written in a foreign language. Do not now look for the answers. They cannot now be given to you because you could not live them. It is a question of experiencing everything. At present, you need to live the question. Perhaps you will gradually, without even noticing it, find yourself experiencing the answer, some distant day."[13]

Welcome to the retreat.

13. Rilke, *Letters to a Young Poet*, 34–35.

PART TWO

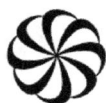

The Retreat

6

Letting the Retreat Unfold

You are in a relationship with God, whether it is something you are actively attending to or not. Through this retreat, I will provide opportunities to engage in that relationship more intentionally. There will be time to reflect on some of the questions and challenges we've discussed and the invitations God is giving us. Also layered into these exercises are some of Baldovin's reasons, which we learned about in part one of the retreat guide, for why we go to mass, such as hearing the Scriptures, having companionship with Christ, and sharing our needs with God. This retreat is not a substitute for communal prayer or the sacrament of the Eucharist, nor a substitute for support groups or therapy. It does provide ways to pray and be with God while walking through this valley.

The time we spend living with dementia can become a profound source of reflection on all of the assumptions we make about what it means to be a human being, what it means to be a Christian, and what it means to be loved by God. As you work through your questions and share them and your concerns with God, as you pray and ask for help, and as you become more intentional about your time with God, it can help nourish your relationship and give you strength for the journey through the Valley of Dementia.

This retreat is a series of exercises to help you explore your spirituality. Benedictine nun Joan Chittister defines spirituality as "the conscious turning of the mind and the spirit to God; that softens the edges of the heart, that increases your understanding, and enlightens your heart."[1] Little by little, be attentive to yourself and to God. Let yourself be where you are in the journey, and let God soften the edges of your heart and life.

Take this retreat at your own pace, or better yet, go at God's pace. Invite God to join you and to guide you. Invite your authentic self to show up. And let the Holy Spirit guide your attention and focus. It might work for you to make some of the exercises a daily practice or weekly, or possibly you work with one per month. You might modify the practices, do them in a different order, or do one exercise repeatedly and skip another. That is all fine. I recommend that you be intentional about setting aside time to journey with God throughout this Valley of Dementia, with all of its twists and turns, good days and bad days. Trust. God is with you, and so are my prayers.

Note that some exercises are available for you to listen to online. These exercises will have an asterisk (*) in the title. The link to the online retreat materials is in the additional resources section.

---

1. Chittister, *Monastic Heart*, 69.

7

Retreat Exercises

EXERCISE ONE | WELCOME BREATH*

I was once assigned a task to spend more time in nature every day. I was feeling overwhelmed and unsure how to accomplish this task, so I decided, somewhat flippantly, to march outside, touch the tree in my backyard, and march back into the house every day. Task completed. The funny thing is, after weeks and months of this. It worked. I began to feel more connected to the land I was living on. I began to want to spend more time outside by that tree.

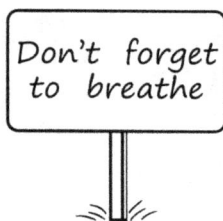

Like walking to the tree, this exercise is simple. I invite you to take one simple deep breath. On the inhale, notice where you are. What room are you in? What objects do you see? Are there others with you? On the exhale, say aloud or to yourself, "Welcome," as you invite yourself to be present and you invite the awareness of God's presence. Repeat as necessary.

> *[God] makes [the] sun rise on the bad*
> *and the good, and causes rain to fall on*
> *the just and the unjust (Matt 5:45 NAB).*
> *However we succeed or fail as a care partner*
> *today, God will be with us, loving us.*

EXERCISE TWO | RITUAL—THE FOUNDATION STONE

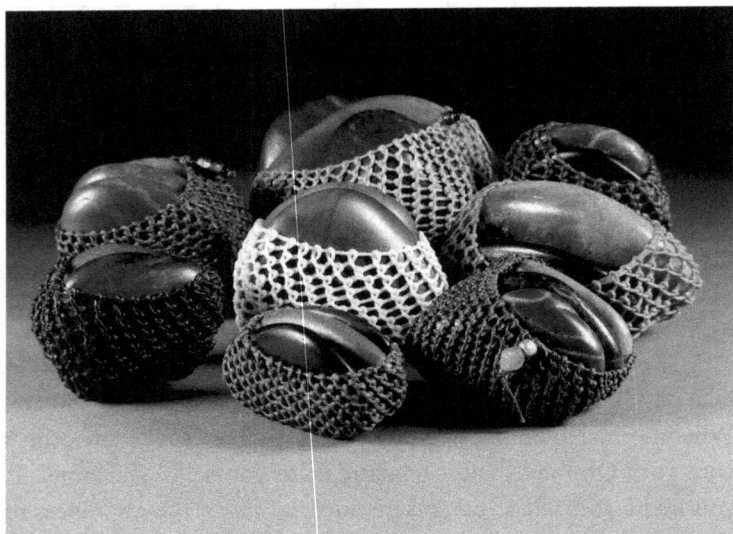

"Together Stones" by Therese Fisher. Stone and waxed linen.

As you embark on this retreat, I invite you to go outside and find a small stone that can fit in the palm of your hand and in your pocket. Carry it with you for the duration of this retreat, or keep it somewhere you can touch or see it regularly. I ask you to remember two things when you touch this rock.

First, God created this rock long before God created you and the person you are care partnering with. And this stone will exist long after you and your care partner have left your bodies. Let it be a symbol of both the longevity and the temporality of human life.

Let it be a reminder of the steadfastness and strength of God, who was present before dementia came into your life, is present now, and will be present after your PLwD has gone home to be with God.

Second, notice the shape of the rock. Is it round but not perfectly round? Is it triangular, but not a perfect triangle? Is it smooth but not perfectly smooth? Whatever its shape and texture, God created this rock, just like God created you. We are all far from perfect. We have smooth parts and rough parts. Our bodies might not be the perfect shape. We certainly do not always make the best decisions or ideal choices. Take a look at your rock again. This rock is one of the joys of God's creation, just like you.

Remember your rock whenever something goes wrong or is not how you want it to be or when you are tired and worn out. Remember that God created it and saw that it was good, just like God created you and sees you as good (Gen 1:31).

EXERCISE THREE | GRATITUDE MOMENT

The Dalai Lama and Archbishop Des-
mond Tutu cite gratitude as one of the
eight pillars of joy. They say, "Gratitude
is the recognition of all that holds us in
the web of life."[1] In this sense, gratitude
can help alleviate our sense of isolation
as we actively engage with the world
around us.

Think about this past week. Write
out three to five things that brought you
a sense of comfort or a sense of peace, however big or small. Take
a moment to thank God for these gifts.

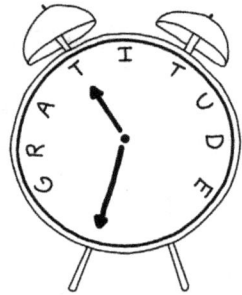

1.

2.

3.

4.

5.

1. Dalai Lama XIV et al., *Book of Joy*, 242.

EXERCISE FOUR | GUIDED MEDITATION—
CONNECTED HEART*

This guided meditation is designed for you to reflect on the physicality of your being, a being that God created and breathed life into
(Gen 2:7). It will help you connect more deeply with your body, your heart, and the heart of God. The meditation takes about twenty minutes and can be modified for shorter or longer periods.

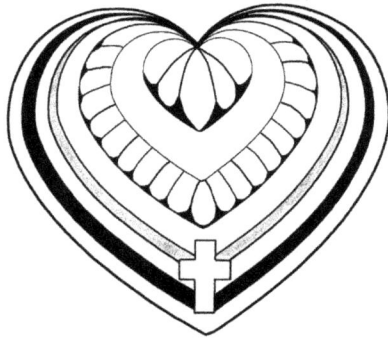

Get in a comfortable position with as few external distractions as possible. Close your eyes, take a few deep breaths, and invite the awareness of God's presence to enter your heart. In this meditation, you will bring attention to parts of your body. As you do, imagine a thread of light connecting that part of your body to your heart, and say aloud or to yourself: "My [name the part of the body you are focusing on] is connected to my heart, which is connected to the heart of God." Notice if there are any shifts in your body as you do this. You might feel peace, relaxation, a tingling sensation, or even a bolt of electricity.

Begin with the top of the head and move down towards your heart, drawing threads of light from your brain, eyes, ears, nose and sinus cavities, lips, mouth, jaw, throat, and neck, all to your heart and to the heart of God. Move down to your shoulders, hands, wrists, forearms, elbows, and upper arm. Drawing a thread from each part to your heart and then from your heart to the Sacred Heart, the heart of God. Then, move to your feet and work your way back up to your heart. Move through your feet, ankles, lower legs, knees, upper legs, hips, pelvic floor, belly, rib cage, chest, and spine.

Once you have completed this, continue to sit and breathe, noticing the sensations in your body. If something is drawing your attention, breathe into that area and again draw a line from that location to your heart and the heart of God. When you are ready, thank God for being part of every part of your being, and slowly return from the meditation and open your eyes.

Now, spend a few minutes journaling about your experience.

_____

_____

_____

_____

_____

EXERCISE FIVE | REFLECT AND JOURNAL— CORE VALUES

Often, as care partners, we have to make choices between things that we should not have to. For example, we should not have to choose between telling an anxious and distressed PLwD for the thirty-seventh time that day that they are home/safe and stepping away for a few minutes to use the restroom. We should not have to choose between letting dinner burn on the stove or letting a PLwD soil themselves.

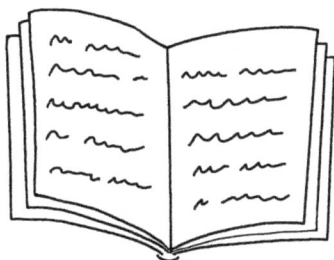

Sometimes, when you have an awareness of your core values, it can help in these situations. It doesn't make the difficult choice go away, but having an awareness of our values allows us to be a little kinder to ourselves in less-than-ideal times. Instead of only seeing the bad choices, we can see the good we are trying to do and the compassion we are trying to bring to a situation, even when we leave them unresolved or undone. It also helps us to be more aware of when our choices are moving us away from what we truly value.

Take some time to journal about what is most important to you. Is it family, God, compassion, service? See if you can identify your top five core values. (If you are struggling with identifying your values, you can do an internet search for "personal values assess-ment" or "core values exercise," and you will find lists of values and other resources to help.)

_____

_____

_____

_____

_____

EXERCISE SIX | PRAYER IN ACTION— FEEDING GOD'S PEOPLE*

We often want God to bless us and bring us instant relief or healing. Less often do we seek to have God work through us. Being overworked and stressed, we usually want God to cut us some slack and fix things right now. These prayer-in-action activities are not about adding more tasks to your day. They are about recognizing the profound love and compassion that can be present in care partnering and inviting God to work through us as we become more attentive to God in what we are already doing. They begin with a short reflection and then an invitation to carry that with you as you go about your day, letting your attentiveness to God transform your acts of care partnering into acts of intentional prayer.

Reflection:

Choose a quiet, comfortable place for this reflection. Begin by taking a few deep breaths to center yourself and prepare your heart and mind for the exercise. Invite the awareness of God's presence to arise within you and invite God to give you new insights into your role as a care partner.

Read and reflect on who Jesus is and what he is doing, as well as who the disciples are and what they are doing in the following passage:

> Taking [the disciples] with him, he retreated to the town of Bethsaida where they could be by themselves. But when the crowd found out, they followed him. Jesus welcomed the crowd and spoke to them about the reign

of God, and healed all who were in need of healing. As sunset approached, the Twelve came and said to Jesus, "Dismiss the crowd, so they can go into the surrounding villages and countryside and find lodging and food, for this is a remote and isolated area." Jesus answered them, "Give them something to eat yourselves!" The disciples replied, "We have nothing but five loaves and two fish. Or do you want us to go and buy food for all these people?" There were about five thousand gathered. Jesus said to the disciples, "Have them sit down in groups of fifty or so." They did so and got them all seated. Then, taking the five loaves and two fishes, Jesus raised his eyes to heaven, said a blessing over them, broke them and gave them to the disciples for distribution to the crowd. They all ate until they were satisfied and, when the leftovers were collected, there were twelve baskets full. (Luke 9:10b–17 TIB)

Jot down any notes from your initial reading of the passage.

_____

_____

_____

_____

_____

Reread the passage, reflecting on the act of feeding (or assisting with feeding) a PLwD, and consider the parallels between your role as a care partner and the compassion and care Jesus showed in the miracle. Ask God how the act of feeding is an expression of God's love. How is what you do similar to Jesus' act of providing food for the masses? How is your role as a care partner similar to that of the disciples? Take some time to journal about this.

_____

44

_____

_____

_____

_____

Reread the passage again and notice if God is inviting you into a new way of approaching your role as a care partner. What do you sense? Is there an invitation? If so, what is it? What is your response to the invitation?

_____

_____

_____

_____

_____

Close the reflection time with a prayer, expressing your feelings and intentions, and asking for patience and generosity or whatever else you need in your role as a care partner.

_____

_____

_____

_____

_____

Taking It with You:

Here are some ways to incorporate this reflection into feeding someone.

- Before you begin feeding the PLwD, have a moment of gratitude and say to yourself, "I am grateful for the opportunity to care for [this person] and provide nourishment."

- While feeding the PLwD, visualize yourself as one of the disciples in the story, offering nourishment and care with love and compassion.

- As you feed the PLwD, pray silently or aloud, "God, as I feed [this person], may your love and compassion flow through me," or "Bless this meal, and may it bring comfort and strength," or some other prayer of your choosing.

- Continue to feed the PLwD with a sense of reverence, mindful of your actions' profound spiritual significance.

- After the meal, take a moment to reflect on what you have just done. For example, you might acknowledge, "In this act of feeding, I feel a deeper connection to the love and compassion of Jesus."

EXERCISE SEVEN | REFLECT AND JOURNAL—
MADE IN THE IMAGE OF GOD

The book of Genesis tells us we are made in the image of God. But what does that really mean? The Bible tells us all sorts of things about who God is—God is a sanctuary (Isa 8:14), a physician (Luke 4:23), and a friend (Jer 3:4). God is jealous and avenging (Nah 1:2). God is forgiving (Nah 9:17) and also a judge (1 Sam 24:15). God is to be feared (1 Chr 16:25). God is a role model (Prov 19:21). These are but a few glimpses into who God is. God's character is complex and sometimes seems contradictory. Who is God for you, and how is that reflected in your life and in your role as a care partner?

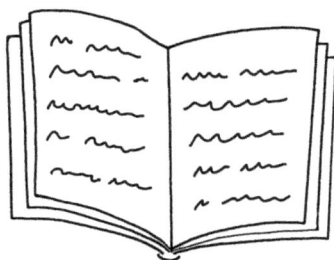

_____

_____

_____

_____

_____

Part Two: The Retreat

"Humankind was created as God's reflection: in the divine image God created them."—Genesis 1:27 TIB

EXERCISE EIGHT | GRATITUDE MOMENT

Gratitude is a way of acknowledging everything "that has made it possible to have the life that we have and the moment that we are experiencing."[2] It is essential to recognize the realities of our challenges. It is also important to acknowledge the gifts we have received. It is not one or the other but both that bring us into the richness of the moment. Because we tend to think about life's challenges quite readily, it is vital to consciously set aside time to attend to gratitude.

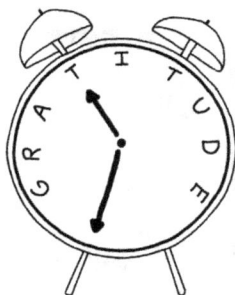

Invite the Holy Spirit to guide your attention to things of beauty you have experienced. List three to five things this week (or in your lifetime) that struck you as beautiful, and take a moment to thank God for allowing you to experience each of them.

1.

2.

3.

4.

5.

2. Dalai Lama XIV et al., *Book of Joy*, 242.

EXERCISE NINE | PRAYING OUTSIDE—
EXPLORING SACRED GROUND

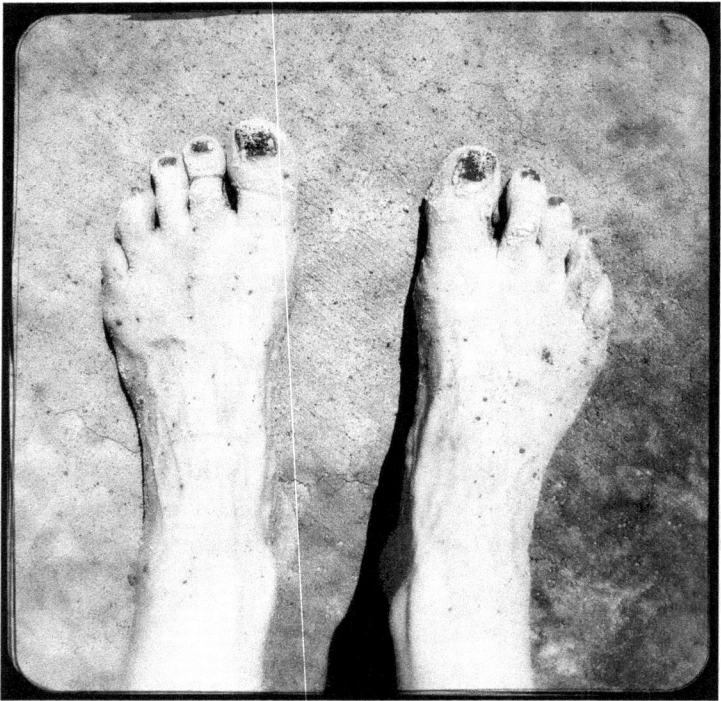

God said to Moses, "Come no nearer! Remove the sandals from your feet, for the place where you stand is holy ground" (Exod 3:5 NAB). Why was the ground sacred? Because God was present. You might not experience the sound of God's voice telling you to take off your shoes. Still, the ground you are walking, the Valley of

Dementia, is holy ground. Jeremiah 23:23–24 tells us that God is everywhere. That means God was present in this valley before you got here and is present with you now. Do not wonder if God is here with you; expect to find God here with you. Go outside to feel the ground and God's creation and presence. If it is safe, remove your shoes and feel the sacred earth and God's presence pressing against your feet and supporting them. Ask for God to reveal God's self to you as you explore the sacred ground around you. Journal about the experience when you return.

_____

_____

_____

_____

_____

EXERCISE TEN | REFLECT AND JOURNAL— SHIFTING FOCUS*

Take a few deep breaths and invite the awareness of God's presence to be known to you. Notice if you sense any shifts when you do so. Ask God to guide you in this exercise and draw your attention to how your life focus has shifted since you became a care partner. In your journaling space, take some time to reflect and answer the following questions.

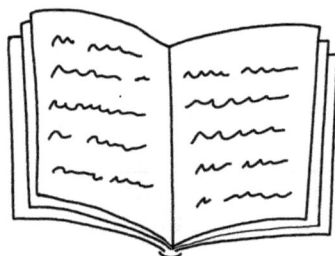

1. What have you given up or diverted your attention from in order to be a care partner?

_____

_____

_____

_____

_____

2. How has this affected your life?

_____

_____

_____

_____

_____

3. What gifts has this change brought you?

_____

_____

_____

_____

_____

4. Ask God, is there anything that you let go of that you need to attend to or refocus on? If not, thank God for the gift of this release. If yes, ask God to breathe love into that area and to show you if there is any specific action you need to take.

_____

_____

_____

_____

_____

5. Take a few minutes to thank God for being with you and sharing this journey with you.

_____

_____

_____

_____

_____

Feel free to return to this exercise as often as it feels fruitful. There might be more than one area of your life that God wants you to look at. Also, ask God if God would like you to revisit any particular area of your life. There might be more that God wants to show you.

> *"Contemplation of the will of God—what it is; what, specifically, you hear it saying to you at this moment—is the ground of the spiritual life."*[3]*—Joan Chittister*

---

3. Chittister, *Monastic Heart*, 69.

EXERCISE ELEVEN | GUIDED
MEDITATION—GOD IN THE SENSES*

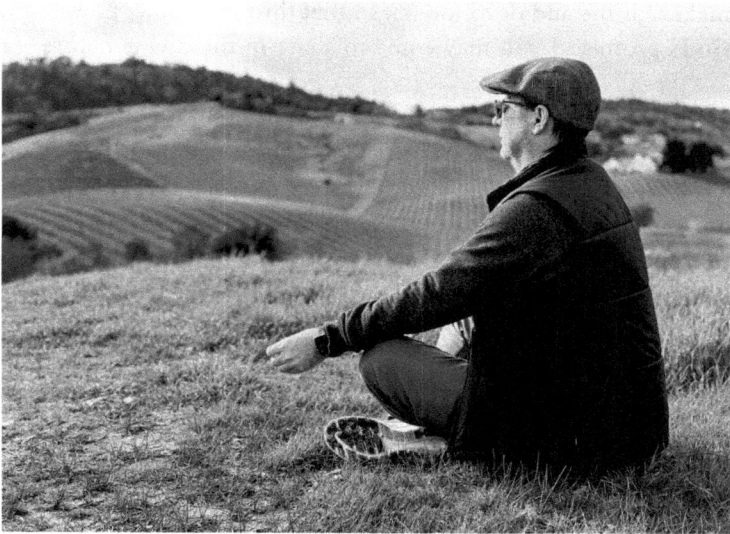

This meditation is designed for you to reflect on your senses and how God is an integral part of who you are. God created you (Gen 1:27). God's law is written in your heart and mind (Heb 10:16). Take this time to contemplate your senses, how you experience the world, and how God is a part of that. It is as if our bodies are designed to know and experience God with and through each of our senses.

Find a comfortable place with as few external distractions as possible. Invite the awareness of God's presence to be with you. It might be helpful to think of a phrase or word that will serve as that invitation for you. During the meditation, if you find yourself getting distracted, use your key phrase to invite the awareness of God's presence to be with you again and return your focus to your breath.

Take a few long, deep breaths. Breathe in and let the noise of the day fall away. Let the "corruption of the world" (2 Pet 1:4) be released from your body. Take another breath and welcome yourself to be fully present and aware of God's presence.

Now, take a few breaths, focusing your attention on the area of your brain, pondering that God's law is written there and that God's "divine power has bestowed on [your mind] everything that makes for life and devotion . . . so that through [God's power and God's promises] you may come to share in the divine nature" (2 Pet 1:3–4 NAB).

The essence of the law written on your mind is found in Jesus' words: "You shall love the Lord your God with all your heart, with all your soul, and with all your mind. . . . You shall love your neighbor as yourself" (Matt 22:37, 39 NAB). These words and God's love to empower them are inescapably a part of your mind. Your mind is designed to grow and share in divine nature.

Now, take a few breaths, focusing your attention on the area of your heart, pondering that God's law is also written there and that God's "divine power has bestowed on [your heart] everything that makes for life and devotion . . . so that through [God's power and God's promises] you may come to share in the divine nature" (2 Pet 1:3–4 NAB).

Imagine the essence of these words fully integrated into your heart: "Love one another. As I have loved you, so you also should love one another." (John 13:34 NAB). These words and God's love to empower them are inescapably a part of your heart. Your heart is formed to grow and share in love and in divine nature.

And so, your senses, which combine the experience of your heart and mind, are also infused with the power of God. Invite God to expand your awareness of your senses and how they enable you to experience, grow, and share in divine nature. As you continue through this exploration of senses, if you experience a lack within a particular sense, it is okay. God is working there, too.

Allow God to draw your attention to how God is working through, for example, a sight impairment or an inability to hear, or invite God to draw your attention to another sense, perhaps even one that is unique to you.

Take a deep breath, focusing your awareness on your eyes. Your eyes take in many sights and information, both joyful and horrific, in person and through media like television, books, computers, and movies. Notice how your eyes, through all of that input, have the innate ability to see God's love around you and in the world.

Take a deep breath, focusing on your ears and the sounds that come into your body. How did God design your ears to love? Can you hear the sound of laughter? The sound of someone crying out? The sound of birthday candles being blown out? How else does your body take in sound? Do you feel the vibration of the sound of a sigh? Where is God entering your life through sound? How is God showing you God's will through the sounds around you? How is God using the sounds you make to bring God's love into the world?

Take a breath now and focus on your nose and your sinus passages. What aspects of God are entering your life through scent? Is it the smell of freshly baked cookies or newly picked flowers? Is it through the smell of your best friend's shampoo or maybe burning incense? How is God using your ability to smell to speak to you? Is the scent of urine how God tells you to tend to those in need? How can you use scent to share God's love in the world?

Take some breaths now, focusing on the area of your mouth. Breathe in and out of your mouth. The very breath of God flows in and through our bodies. How is God revealing God's self to you and others through the mouth and taste? God's law is within us, so we can know and taste it. Every word we utter has the potential to speak God's love and to taste of God's sweetness. How is God using your mouth to allow you to sense God's love and to give others the sense of God's love?

Now, take some deep breaths and focus your attention on your hands and the feel of your skin. How is God using the sensations of your skin to reveal God's will? Are you sharing God's love with a wave, a handshake, or holding a baby? How does the way your skin feels reveal the presence of God? Do you feel a shiver when you hear God's word? Do you feel the vibration of God's love? Do you lift your hands in praise?

Take some time now to thank God for creating you with everything you need to experience God, to enact God's law, and to share in the divine nature.

Dear God, you have created us and designed us to be vessels of your love. Because we forget, you wrote your laws on our hearts and on our minds within the very essence of who we are. Enliven our senses so that we may see, hear, smell, taste, and even touch your love. Help us to be fully alive as the beings you created us to be. Amen.

Take some time to journal about your experience.

_____

_____

_____

_____

_____

EXERCISE TWELVE | PRAYING OUTSIDE—
SEEING GOD IN THE WORLD

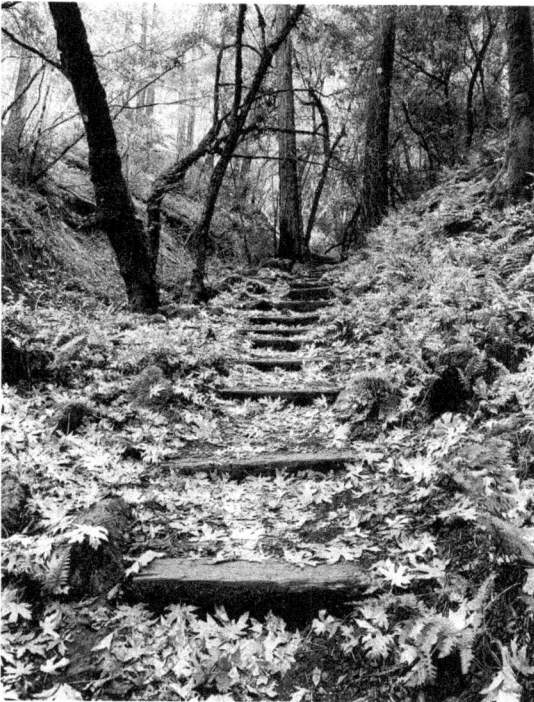

While the PLwD might lose the peripheral vision in their eyes, care partners can also lose their peripheral vision for life outside their current circumstances. This exercise is to go outside and see the essence of the world around you. If you are able to, spend about thirty minutes walking or simply being outside. If thirty minutes is too long, give yourself three minutes or even thirty seconds. Just be intentional.

Invite the awareness of God's presence within you and ask God to show you God's presence in the world around you. Notice what God draws your attention to; when your focus lands on something, notice that God is in this, too.

Each time you encounter something, that which you encounter offers an image or a testimony of God. What does God look like? What does God sound like? What does God smell like? I find it helpful to say to myself as I walk, for example, "God is in the street. God is in the power line. God is in the dried leaf. God is in the gum wrapper." In this way, I acknowledge God's presence in all things. If nothing can separate us from the love of God (Rom 8:38–39), could it also mean that *everything* is a path through which we can find God? Make some notes about your experience.

_____

_____

_____

_____

_____

EXERCISE THIRTEEN | RITUAL—REMEMBERING COMMUNITY (OR STICKY NOTE FRIENDS)

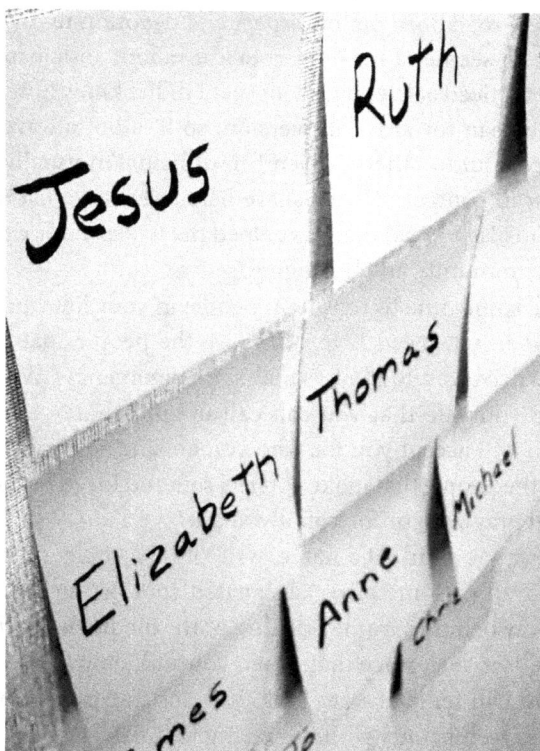

One would think that after living through the arrival of the CO-VID-19 pandemic, we all might be experts at navigating isolation and how to find meaningful connections. It would seem, however, that we are still quite skilled at feeling alone, misunderstood, and unsure where to turn.

Even before her official diagnosis, the day my stepmom began having significant symptoms was the day her dying process began for me. Because of my background, I knew the trajectory. Her death, even though it hasn't happened yet, has been a palpable part of my experience of her life. So, for me, her decline has been agonizing. Not wanting to push my family members into my stage of pain and grief, I kept my feelings to myself. Instead, I chose to hold space for their unique experiences and optimism. It was a long, lonely road born out of respect and devotion to my family.

Once it seemed time to start talking about anticipatory grief, I was so practiced at keeping silent that I didn't know how to begin. I generally lean towards introversion, so it is not always easy for me to reach out to others. When I need help, I'm usually at a loss for whom to contact. What I share here, creating a list of "sticky note friends," is a ritual that has helped me to feel a more profound sense of community and belonging.

Take some time to reflect on people in your life who you can call on when you need help. Who are the people that would be willing to drive you to the hospital in an emergency? Who are the people in your life that you can call up and share your feelings with, who will accept you for who you are and not try to fix you? Who are the people that make you feel safe and loved? Who do you know will pray with or for you if you ask?

When you think of a name, write it on a sticky note and put it on the wall or some other designated spot. It can be visible or tucked away behind a framed picture or the medicine cabinet door. It just needs to be a place that, when you suddenly find yourself at a loss, you will remember to look. It is an "in case of emergency, break glass" setup, only without having to break glass.

It doesn't matter how many you have. I feel abundantly blessed to have just a few. Maybe you have one, or perhaps you have hundreds. (If you are having trouble getting started, make God your first sticky note friend.) When you need help, go to that spot where your sticky note friends are and remind yourself who they are and that they care. Then, reach out to one of them.

I have walked to the wall many times to look at those names, occasionally only to remind myself that there are people in the world who care about me, and I can call if I need to. Remembering that I have a community of friends has been tremendously helpful. Also helpful is intentionally reaching out to these individuals regularly. Even if it is just a text to say hello, tending to the threads that connect us is a practice of honoring our community.

Don't feel like you need a complete list all at once. It took me months to create my list, which continues to evolve. People's sticky notes come down, and others go up on the wall as life shifts. It's okay. They never need to know. It's your list, and you can keep it somewhere private.

It is not always easy to reach out to others when you are feeling isolated. For some, just seeing this list will bring comfort. For others, you might want to reach out but don't know what to say. Here are some ways you can add to this practice by reaching out:

- Ask a sticky note friend to send you jokes to cheer you up.

- Call a sticky note friend, tell them you really want to hear a friendly voice, and ask them if they will tell you about what is going on in their life while you sit and listen.

- If you do not feel like a conversation but still want to connect, ask if you can just sit together in silent prayer or meditation for a little while. This works in person and also works well on video calls.

- Ask a sticky note friend to pray for you. You can be as vulnerable or as vague as you feel comfortable. I once asked all my friends to pray for something I had written on a piece of paper in an envelope because I didn't want to tell them what it was about. I kept the envelope in my special prayer space at home. I felt the love and support that came with those prayers and honored my privacy.

- Reach out to your sticky note friends and ask them if there is something you can pray for on their behalf (if you do not want to focus on what is going on for you right now but want to make a connection).

- Consider saying yes when your sticky note friends ask if they can help. If you don't have anything specific you need help with, ask them to liaise with God for you. Maybe today you ask your friends to love God for you because you are so angry at God for this painful situation that you don't even want to speak to God right now. Or, ask them to have hope for you because you don't feel it right now. Or, ask them to believe that you will get through this. You know what is missing in your life and your relationship with God.

- I repeat, let them help. If you do not want to engage in a spiritual conversation, ask them to pick you up something from the grocery store or recommend a good book. If your goal is to make a connection, it does not matter what you ask them for; what matters is that you reach out. Knowing they care enough to bring you a loaf of bread, extra toilet paper, or whatever will feel nourishing. You can also make a list of things that people can help you with, even if right now is not when you need the help. If someone asks, you can review the list and see if anything would be a good match for them. Your list can include everything from sitting with the PLwD so you can go out for a walk to funeral planning, from bringing you flowers to helping you clean the kitchen. Consider saying "thank you" when they help and letting them know how their help impacted you.

- Call a sticky note friend and be honest about what you want. For example, you could say, "Hey, I'm feeling really angry and upset today, and I need to vent. Do you have a few minutes? I won't be rational; don't try to correct me, fix me, or solve the situation. I just need you to listen, okay?" (Remember, they are a sticky note friend because you trust them and they support you.)

- Set up a regular schedule to connect. It could be for tea, a short walk, or a phone call once a month on a specific day or even daily at a particular time, with the understanding that if things come up, you can reschedule. Having that item on the calendar in the future helps you remember you are not alone now and you won't be alone in the future.

EXERCISE FOURTEEN | PRAYER— CRY OUT TO GOD*

Care partnering with someone living with dementia can be a challenging and emotionally taxing journey. This retreat exercise is meant to provide you with a space for self-expression, for connecting more deeply with God and your faith, and for finding solace in your role as a care partner. Remember that having complex and contradictory emotions is normal. And it is okay to have them about God. Turning to God in moments of distress, anger, or confusion is a sign of strength and faith. It is an acknowledgment of your relationship with God and trust in God.

You will use excerpts from one of the laments in the book of Psalms as a starting point for this personal reflection and prayer. According to Walter Bruggemann in *From Whom No Secrets Are Hid*, one of the many gifts the Psalms offers us is this gift of disclosure.[4] Praying the Psalms gives us a chance to cry out to God and to tell God everything: what we fear or are angry about, our worries, and even our praise. And, as Pennebaker reminds us, keeping secrets is bad for our health. It is physically demanding and negatively influences our short and long-term biological and mental health.[5] Use this exercise as an opportunity to give God those secrets that you have been holding on to.

Find a quiet and comfortable place with as few distractions as possible. Begin by taking a few deep breaths to center yourself and calm your mind. Invite yourself to be completely honest with God.

---

4. Brueggemann, *From Whom No Secrets*, xiii–xxiv.
5. Pennebaker and Smyth, *Opening Up by Writing It Down*, 10.

Invite the awareness of the presence of God to arise within you and invite God to hear what is on your heart.

Read these verses from Psalm 13 as a starting point for your reflection:

> How long, O Lord? Will you forget me forever? How long will you hide your face from me? How long must I wrestle with my thoughts and day after day have sorrow in my heart? How long will my enemy triumph over me? Look on me and answer, O Lord my God. Give light to my eyes, or I will sleep in death, and my enemy will say, 'I have overcome him,' and my foes will rejoice when I fall. (Ps 13:1–4 NIV)

Take a moment to meditate on these verses, considering your own situation as a care partner. Reflect on your feelings, challenges, and the emotions you carry within.

Now, complete these verses in your own words, expressing your thoughts and feelings to God:

"How long, Lord? I feel . . ."

_____

_____

_____

_____

_____

"How long must I wrestle with my thoughts about . . ."

_____

_____

_____

_____

_____

"Look on me and answer, my God. I seek your guidance in . . ."

_____

_____

_____

_____

_____

"Give light to my eyes, so that I may find hope and strength to . . ."

_____

_____

_____

_____

After completing these sentences, take a moment to sit in silence and allow any additional thoughts, feelings, needs, or hopes to surface. Share them with God.

_____

_____

_____

_____

_____

Conclude your reflection with an acknowledgment of who God is for you:

"God, to me, you are . . ."

_____

_____

_____

_____

_____

"I trust in your . . ."

_____

_____

_____

_____

_____

"I am grateful for your . . ."

_____

_____

_____

_____

_____

Close with your own prayer, offering your concerns, gratitude, and desires to God.

EXERCISE FIFTEEN | REFLECT AND JOURNAL— RELEASING THE BURDEN OF HOPE

I recently attended a talk by author and psychologist Ayelet Gundar-Goshen. She spoke about her work assisting people with their trauma after the Hamas attack in October of 2023.[6] She shared a story about someone grieving the loss of their mother, who was killed in the attack. That person said that they were grateful their mother had died so they could begin to mourn her loss instead of languishing in the pain of hoping she might still be out there. Sometimes, the grief of death seems far more straightforward, even easier somehow, than the hopes that we feel obligated to hold on to. In situations like this, it is instinctual to hold out hope for the return of lost loved ones until there is absolute proof that they are gone.

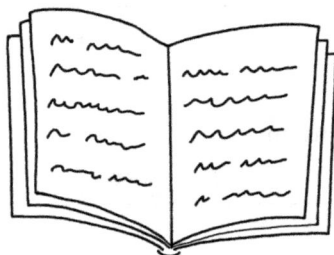

This story reminds me of what it is like to be a care partner, searching for proof that the PLwD is still with us, the person we know and love. In our efforts to embrace their life, we often stumble upon hope. We hope they will remember us, that they still love us, and that they will get better. Living with the hope that they will return to us can be excruciating. At times, some of us long to lay down this burdensome hope when our loved one dies at long last.

6. Gundar-Goshen, "Trauma: A Conversation."

Burdensome hope is the kind of hope focused on what we want and think will fill the void in us. It is a kind of hope limited by how we see and understand the word. The treasured things we hope for can become attachments that keep us from being fully alive. Take some time today to journal about what hope you are holding on to. What are those sweet and precious things you long for? Are you hoping to hear "I love you," "thank you," or how you have made a difference in your care partner's life? Are you hoping to hear them laugh again, tell a story, see them dance, or maybe tell you they are sorry? Take time today to tell God what is in your heart, all the hopes weighing you down. What are the hopes you are afraid to hope or know you should not hope? What are the hopes you are embarrassed to tell anyone? Give them to God.

"Dear God, what I hope for the most right now is . . ."

_____

_____

_____

_____

_____

Is there anything that God is hoping for you?

_____

_____

_____

_____

_____

EXERCISE SIXTEEN | GIVING HOPE; CREATING A LEGACY

Review your journal from yesterday and highlight the keywords of the things you told God you have been hoping for. Take some time today to reflect on those things. Is there any way that you can take what you hoped for and turn it into a gift for someone else? In his book *Finding Meaning: The Sixth Stage of Grief*, David Kessler recommends taking your grief and channeling that energy into creating a legacy.[7] This helps us to find meaning in our grief. You don't need to wait for the person you are care partnering with to die before you begin to celebrate their life and your relationship by turning it into a legacy. You can start small.

Here are some examples: If you long to see your loved one smile again, can you, in their honor, smile at someone today? If you wish they remembered who you are, can you go out today and meet someone new and learn a little about who they are? Or can you call a friend and learn something new about them? If you wish the PLwD would apologize for something they did to you, can you find someone in your life who you've been less than perfect with and apologize to them? If you wish that the PLwD's life

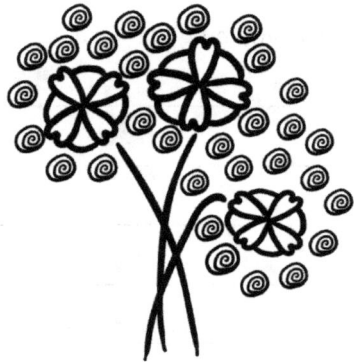

7. Kessler, *Finding Meaning*, 206–18.

wasn't dragging on so long, can you reach out to someone who is grieving and comfort them?

Decide one small thing you will do to begin creating a legacy.

"Today I will . . ."

_____

_____

_____

_____

_____

> *"A generous person will prosper; whoever refreshes others will be refreshed."—Proverbs 11:25 NIV*

EXERCISE SEVENTEEN | GRATITUDE MOMENT

Sometimes, it can be hard to think of things to be grateful for. One way to get around this stumbling block is to notice the things you are grateful for not having. For example, "I am grateful that I was not injured when I fell yesterday," "I'm grateful that I didn't get any telemarketing calls this week," or "I'm grateful that I was not hit by a car." Be as creative as you like.

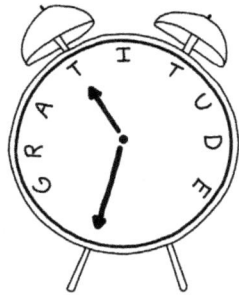

Reflect on the past week. List three to five things you are grateful did not happen. Say a prayer of gratitude for the many graces in your life.

1.

2.

3.

4.

5.

EXERCISE EIGHTEEN | REFLECT AND JOURNAL—RAISING OF THE WIDOW'S SON*

The story of Jesus rais-
ing the widow's son has
always fascinated me as a
care partner, particularly
since I have a substantial
value in asking people's
permission before I do
something with or for
them. As care partners,
we struggle between engaging with the PLwD to do an activity and
doing the action for them. Which choice is safer, faster, easier, and
will give the PLwD the best quality of life? Read the story of the
raising of the widow's son.

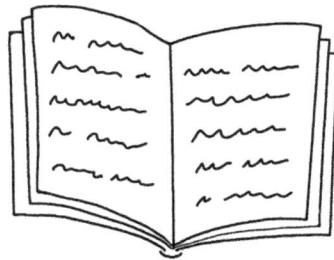

> Soon afterward, Jesus went to a town called Nain, and his
> disciples and a large crowd went along with him. As he ap-
> proached the town gate, a dead person was being carried
> out—the only son of his mother, and she was a widow. And
> a large crowd from the town was with her. When the Lord
> saw her, his heart went out to her and he said, "Don't cry."
> Then he went up and touched the coffin they were carry-
> ing him on, and the bearers stood still. He said, "Young
> man, I say to you, get up!" The dead man sat up and began
> to talk, and Jesus gave him back to his mother. They were
> all filled with awe and praised God. "A great prophet has
> appeared among us," they said. "God has come to help his
> people." This news about Jesus spread throughout Judea
> and the surrounding country. (Luke 7:11–17 NIV)

Do you notice that Jesus does not ask the widow if she wants her son to be raised or if it is okay with her if he does it? There is also no report of asking the dead man's soul if he wants to be alive on earth again. It appears that Jesus is simply compelled to act based on the stirrings in his heart, and so raises the man.

Reread the story more slowly this time. Imagine yourself at the scene. Perhaps you are a part of the large crowd following Jesus, or maybe you are part of the crowd surrounding the widow. What do you notice about the scene? About the people? What are people wearing? What does the ground feel like? Is it hot, or is it cool out? What time of day is it? You see the coffin. What is it made out of? You see Jesus touch it. Watch how the crowd responds. How do you respond? Make some notes about what caught your attention in the scene.

_____

_____

_____

_____

_____

Now that this miracle has taken place, find Jesus. There is a break in the gathering as though God has intended for you to meet Jesus. Approach and ask Jesus how he knew what to do. Did he know what he was doing? Did he make a conscious choice about what was best, and if so, how did he discern what was best for the woman? For the man? Or, did his body just act without consciously thinking things through? Did he know for sure that what he was doing was the will of God? Take some time to journal any responses to these question.

_____

_____

_____

_____

_____

Reread the story one more time. Ask God if there is anything else that God wants to draw your attention to in this story. If so, write about that here.

_____

_____

_____

_____

_____

EXERCISE NINETEEN | PRAYER IN ACTION—BATHING AS A BLESSING*

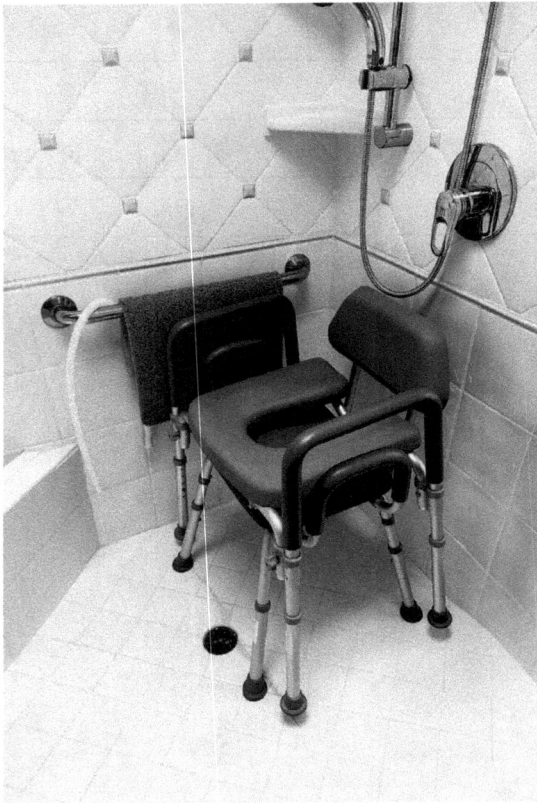

These prayer-in-action activities are not about adding more tasks to your day. They are about recognizing the profound love and compassion that can be present in care partnering with those living with dementia, and inviting God to work through us as we become more attentive to God within the activities we are already doing. They begin with a short reflection and then an invitation to carry that with you as you go about your day, letting your attentiveness to God transform your acts of care partnering into acts of intentional prayer.

Reflection:

Choose a quiet, comfortable place for this reflection. Begin by taking a few deep breaths to center yourself and prepare your heart and mind for the exercise. Invite the awareness of God's presence to arise within you and invite God to give you new insights into your role as a care partner.

Read and reflect on this passage:

> Fully aware that the Father had put everything into his power and that he had come from God and was returning to God, he rose from supper and took off his outer garments. He took a towel and tied it around his waist. Then he poured water into a basin and began to wash the disciples' feet and dry them with the towel around his waist. He came to Simon Peter, who said to him, "Master, are you going to wash my feet?" Jesus answered and said to him, "What I am doing, you do not understand now, but you will understand later." (John 13:3–7 NAB)

Jot down any notes from your initial reading of the passage.

_____

_____

_____

_____

_____

Reread the passage. Reflect on bathing the PLwD as you read, and ask God to show you parallels between your role as a care partner and the love and care Jesus showed in washing the disciples' feet. How is bathing an expression of Jesus' love and compassion? Take some time to reflect and journal.

_____

_____

_____

_____

_____

Reread the passage again and notice if God is inviting you into a new way of approaching your role as a care partner. What do you sense? Is there an invitation? If so, what is it? What is your response to the invitation?

_____

_____

_____

_____

_____

Close the reflection time with a prayer, expressing your feelings and intentions, and asking for patience and generosity or whatever else you need in your role as a care partner.

_____

_____

_____

_____

_____

Taking It with You:

Here are some ways to incorporate this reflection into bathing someone.

- Before you bathe the PLwD, have a moment of gratitude and say to yourself, "I am grateful for the opportunity to tenderly care for [this person] by washing their body."

- While bathing the PLwD, visualize yourself as Jesus in the story, humbly offering this gift to his disciples with love and compassion.

- As you bathe the PLwD, pray silently or aloud, "God, as I wash [this person], may your love and compassion flow through me," or "Bless them, that what they do not need is washed away and may this act bring comfort and health," or some other prayer of your choosing.

- Continue to bathe the PLwD with a sense of reverence and humility, mindful of the moment's tenderness and the profound spiritual significance of your actions.

- After the bathing, take a moment to reflect on what you have just done. For example, you might acknowledge, "In this act of washing, I feel a deeper connection to the love and compassion that Jesus had for his disciples."

EXERCISE TWENTY | REFLECT AND JOURNAL— A SUFFERING GOD

Before Jesus died, he lived with being crucified. He hung on the cross in that liminal space of being both alive and also a dying body. This was an act of solidarity. In your care partnering relationship, you are in solidarity with Christ as you accompany PLwD and Jesus in that liminal space of not quite here and not quite there. Jesus suffered to know our suffering, and we know God more deeply in our suffering. When we trust that God is in our suffering, it changes the nature of our suffering. It moves from feeling like a place void of God to an experience of being in a relationship with God. Ask God to show you where God is amid your suffering. How is God present to you? How is God tending to you? Journal about that here.

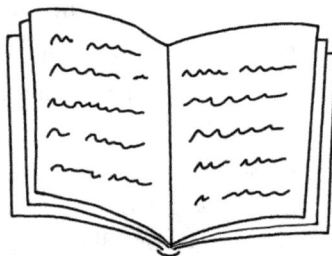

_____

_____

_____

_____

_____

EXERCISE TWENTY-ONE | GRATITUDE MOMENT

Gratitude is a form of rejoicing and people who practice it are less likely to take
life and all of its gifts for granted.[8] By
engaging in these gratitude moments,
you are in essence, strengthening your
gratitude muscles and recalibrating
your life to be more in balance.

Reflect on the past week. Invite
the Holy Spirit to guide your attention
to things that made your role as care
partner easier in some way. List three to five things that supported
you this week as a care partner. They could be objects, people, or
even resources. Take some time to rejoice and say a prayer of gratitude for these tools/gifts.

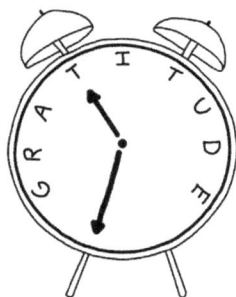

1.

2.

3.

4.

5.

8. Dalai Lama XIV et al., *Book of Joy*, 247.

EXERCISE TWENTY-TWO | PRAYER IN ACTION—HELPING SOMEONE TO DRESS

These prayer-in-action activities are not about adding more tasks to your day. They are about recognizing the profound love and compassion that can be present in care partnering and inviting God to work through us as we become more attentive to God in what we are already doing. They begin with a short reflection and then an invitation to carry that with you as you go about your day, letting your attentiveness to God transform your acts of care partnering into acts of intentional prayer.

Reflection:

Choose a quiet, comfortable place for this reflection. Begin by taking a few deep breaths to center yourself and prepare your heart and mind for the exercise. Invite the awareness of God's presence to arise within you and invite God to give you new insights into your role as a care partner.

Read and reflect on the following passages:

> YHWY made clothes of animal skins for the woman and the man to wear. (Gen 3:21 TIB)

> I gave you a solemn oath and entered into a covenant with you, declares Sovereign YHWH, and you became mine. I bathed you with water, washed the blood from you and anointed you with oil. I gave you brocaded robes and sandals of fine leather. I dressed you in a linen headband and a silk cloak. I adorned you with jewelry—bracelets on your wrists, a chain around your neck, a ring in your

nose, earrings on your ears, and a beautiful diadem on your head. So you were adorned with gold and silver, clothed in fine linen and brocade. (Ezek 16:10 TIB)

For YHWH is the God of gods, the Sovereign of sovereigns, the great God, powerful and awe-inspiring, who has no favorites and cannot be bribed; who brings justice to the orphan and the widowed, and who befriends the foreigner among you with food and clothing. (Deut 10:17–18 TIB)

Jot down any reflections from your initial reading of the passage.

_____

_____

_____

_____

Reread the passages, reflecting on the activity of helping someone get dressed, and consider the parallels between your role as a care partner and God's generosity in clothing us. How is aiding someone to dress an expression of God's love, compassion, and generosity?

_____

_____

_____

_____

_____

Reread the passages again and notice if God is inviting you into a new way of approaching your role as a care partner. What do you sense? Is there an invitation? If so, what is it? What is your response to the invitation?

_____

_____

_____

_____

_____

Close the reflection time with a prayer, expressing your feelings and intentions, and asking for patience and generosity or whatever else you need in your role as a care partner.

_____

_____

_____

_____

_____

Taking It with You:

Here are some ways to incorporate this reflection into dressing someone.

- Before you help dress the PLwD, have a moment of gratitude and say to yourself, "I am grateful for the opportunity to lovingly care for [this person] by clothing them."
- While aiding in clothing the PLwD, visualize yourself there with God, generously dressing God's people, be they Adam

and Eve, God's first human creations, or people generations later. Allow the love and generosity that God has repeated throughout time to be present with you in this moment.

- As you assist in dressing the PLwD, pray silently or aloud, "God, as [this person] is clothed, may your care, attentiveness, and generosity flow through me," or "Bless them that they feel safe, comfortable, and warm," or another prayer of your choosing.

- Continue to assist the PLwD with a sense of reverence, generosity, and care, mindful of the moment's tenderness you are sharing and the sacred significance of your actions as you act in God's image.

- After the person is clothed, take a moment to reflect on what has just taken place. For example, you might acknowledge, "As God clothed us, so we clothe each other in love."

EXERCISE TWENTY-THREE | GUIDED MEDITATION—A GIFT*⁹

Find a comfortable position in a location with as few distractions as possible. Take a few long, deep breaths. Breathe in and allow the breath to flow through your head, clearing away what happened earlier in the day. Take another deep breath and allow it to flow through your heart, reawakening you to your connection with God's love. As you inhale again, let the breath fill your belly, bringing you closer to this moment. If you get distracted at any time, just come back to your breath.

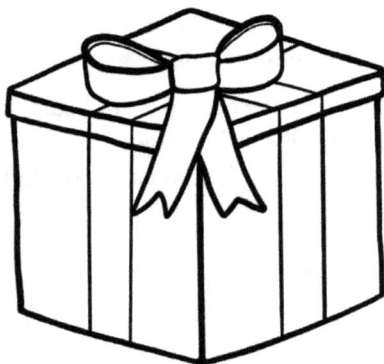

Bring to mind someone you love, someone who cared about you and tended to you when you were struggling or not feeling well. It could be a friend, a family member, a teacher, or a holy being. It could be someone living or someone who has died. Hold them in your consciousness for the length of a few breaths.

Invite them to come and sit in front of you. Maybe reach out and hold their hands for a while. Gaze at them and let them gaze at you. What do you notice about them? Are they smiling? What

9. Based on a meditation I led as part of my coursework for "Mindfulness" (PS 2561: Pastoral Counseling: A Person-Centered Approach to Ministry, Jesuit School of Theology, Berkeley, CA, spring 2022).

look do they have in their eyes? How does their skin feel? Can you hear their breath? Continue to gaze at them, allowing the feelings of your love for each other to grow.

Take a moment to tell them what is going on for you regarding being a care partner. Tell them about the PLwD. Tell them how you are feeling. Notice how they respond as they take in your story. Ask them if they would be willing to give you a gift to help you along this care partnering journey.

Imagine the person lifting their hands up and out towards you as if to offer you something. Looking at their hands, you notice they glow with beautiful, brilliant light. You wonder what this might mean, but you sense it is their gift for you, so you welcome it.

Slowly and gently, they reach over to place their loving hands on a part of your body. The light seems to brighten as it gets closer to you and somehow gets even brighter when they touch you. Notice the part of your body that is being held. Feel the light enter into you, healing, transforming. Allow yourself to receive the light. Does this light have a particular feeling or sense to it? A shape? A taste? A sound? A meaning?

Sit with this for a couple of minutes, being in connection, in communion with this gift. Breathe it in. If you find yourself getting distracted, that's okay. Come on back. You are welcome here, just as you are. Remember again your loved one. They are reaching out to you, holding you, loving you, and gifting you what you need. Take some time to rest in and enjoy this experience.

You will soon begin to return from this visit, so take a moment to acknowledge and thank your loved one for their presence and the gift they shared with you today. You might feel called to tell them you love them. When you feel ready, take another deep breath, open your eyes, and return to the present moment. Take some time to journal about your experience.

EXERCISE TWENTY-FOUR | PRAYING OUTSIDE— WALK IN THE UNITY OF ALL THINGS

Today, I invite you to walk or spend some time outside. Previously, during the retreat, you went outside, noticing God's presence in all things. This time, observe the connectedness of all things. Invite the awareness of God's presence to arise within you. Begin by reading Col 1:16–17 and the Navajo prayer below.

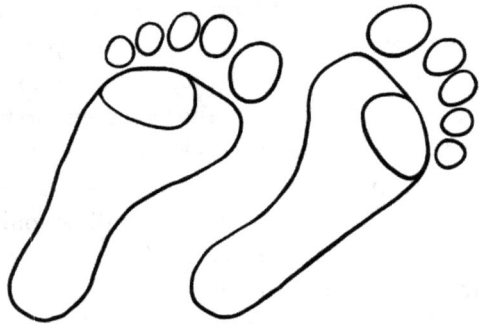

> "The mountains, I become part of it . . .
> The herbs, the fir tree, I become part of it.
> The morning mists, the clouds,
>   the gathering waters,
>   I become part of it.
> The wilderness, the dew drops, the pollen, . . .
> I become part of it."—From a Navajo Prayer[10]

10. Martin, *Way of the Human Being*, 25.

> *"For in Christ were created all things in heaven and on earth: everything visible and invisible, Thrones, Dominations, Sovereignties, Powers—all things were created through Christ and for Christ. Before anything was created, Christ existed, and all things hold together in Christ."—Colossians 1:16–17 TIB*

As you begin your walk, invite God to join you, and then become aware of what God draws your attention to. As you notice each thing, say to yourself, "This [object or being], I am a part of it; we are one [in God]." Keep repeating this for each thing your eye is drawn to during your walk. When you are finished, thank God for blessing you with being a part of God's creation and for everything on this earth that is part of your family.

What did you notice? What is it like to be connected to all things?

_____

_____

_____

_____

_____

EXERCISE TWENTY-FIVE | PRAYER IN ACTION—ASSISTING WITH MOBILITY*

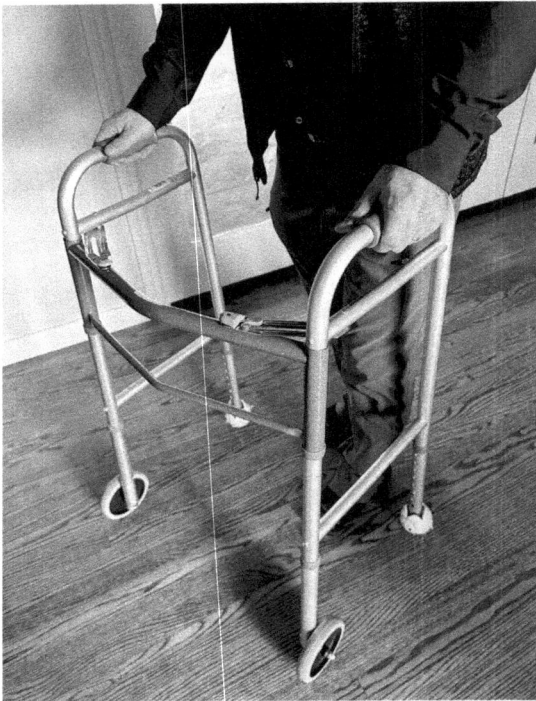

These prayer-in-action activities are not about adding more tasks to your day. They are about recognizing the profound love and compassion that can be present in care partnering and inviting God to work through us as we become more attentive to God in what we are already doing. They begin with a short reflection and then an invitation to carry that with you as you go about your day, letting your attentiveness to God transform your acts of care partnering into acts of intentional prayer.

Reflection:

Choose a quiet, comfortable place for this reflection. Begin by taking a few deep breaths to center yourself and prepare your heart and mind for the exercise. Invite the awareness of God's presence to arise within you and invite God to give you new insights into your role as a care partner.

Read and reflect on the following passage:

> Sometime after this, there was a Jewish festival and Jesus went up to Jerusalem. Now in Jerusalem, near the Sheep Gate, there is a pool with five porticoes; its Hebrew name is Bethesda. The place was crowded with sick people—those who were blind, lame, or paralyzed—lying there waiting for the water to move. An angel of God would come down to the pool from time to time, to stir up the water; the first one to step into the water after it had been stirred up would be completely healed. One person there had been sick for thirty-eight years. Jesus, who knew this person had been sick for a long time, said, "Do you want to be healed?" "Rabbi," the sick one answered, "I don't have anyone to put me into the pool once the water has been stirred up. By the time I get there, someone else has gone in ahead of me." Jesus replied, "Stand up! Pick up your mat and walk."(John 5:1–8 TIB)

Jot down any notes from your initial reading of the passage.

_____

_____

_____

_____

_____

Reread the passage, reflecting on the physicality of helping someone move from lying down to sitting up, from sitting to standing, or walking from one location to another. Consider the parallels between your role as a care partner and Jesus' compassion and care during the miracle of curing the man at Bethesda. How is giving gentle reminders to someone who has forgotten how to use their body an expression of God's love, compassion, and care? How is providing physical support for muscles that are no longer strong enough for independent mobility an expression of God's love?

_____

_____

_____

_____

_____

Reread the passage again and notice if God is inviting you into a new way of approaching your role as a care partner. What do you sense? Is there an invitation? If so, what is it? What is your response to the invitation?

_____

_____

_____

_____

_____

Close the reflection time with a prayer, expressing your feelings and intentions, and asking for patience and generosity or whatever else you need in your role as a care partner.

_____

_____

_____

_____

_____

Taking It with You:

Here are some ways to incorporate this reflection into assisting someone with mobility.

- Before you assist the PLwD, have a moment of gratitude, saying to yourself, "I am grateful for the opportunity to tenderly care for [this person] by helping them to move."

- While assisting the PLwD, visualize yourself as Jesus in the story, humbly offering this gift of mobility to someone who had long been neglected.

- As you assist the PLwD, pray silently or aloud a prayer such as, "God, as I invite mobility for [this person], may your love and compassion flow through me," or "Bless [this person], that their spirit and their love might move freely."

- Continue to assist the PLwD with mobility while holding a sense of reverence and humility, mindful of the moment's tenderness, generosity, and the profound spiritual significance of your actions.

- After assisting them, take a moment to reflect on what you have just done. For example, you might acknowledge, "In this act of mobility, I feel a deeper connection to the love and compassion that Jesus had for those that struggle with mobility and for those society has neglected."

EXERCISE TWENTY-SIX | RITUAL PREPARATION—LETTING GO OF THE PERFECT DEATH[11]

Perfectionism is rampant in our culture. Many of us try to be flawless, get perfect grades, make the most exquisite meal, give the best gift, and have the ideal body. We try to be the perfect employee, friend, child, spouse, or parent. Care partners are not exempt from this desire. We try to get things right and give the PLwD the perfect life, or at least as close to it as possible. We even sometimes try to create for them the perfect death based on our own needs and desires or those shared with us by the PLwD. This ritual is a little more involved than the other exercises. So, give yourself time to reflect and pray on the recipe and gather its "ingredients." I've broken it down into two stages. This exercise is the planning stage, and the next exercise is enacting the ritual. It doesn't have to be perfect. Remember that God's grace is sufficient, and God's power is made perfect in weakness (2 Cor 12:9).

The letting go of the perfect death ritual is inspired by my own experience of being a care partner for my stepmom. I wanted dearly to give her the perfect death because she gave so much to me. It is the least I could do, right? I know better. I was trained on the principles of hospice in 2008 by Providence Hospice in Portland, Oregon. They are: know your role, know what your role is

---

11. Based on a ritual I performed as part of my coursework for "Letting Go of the Perfect Death: A Ritual" (FT 8251: Making Rituals Rich, San Francisco Theological Seminary, San Anselmo, CA, spring 2023).

not, it is not your death, it is not your family, you do not have to fix it, you are part of a team, and listen, listen, listen.[12]

These beautiful guiding principles fell apart when I realized it *was* my family. My role is different now and not clearly defined. Is it a knowledgeable end-of-life care partner, daughter, experienced Alzheimer's care partner, spiritual coach, or nursing assistant? My role has jumped in and out of all of these. As her illness has progressed, many of these roles have been "taken over" by people on her professional caregiving team, leaving me with less and less to do for her and more and more feelings of helplessness. I was carrying on my shoulders a notion that every bit of my life had trained me for this moment, and I was going to see to it that she had a good death!

And then the hospice principles came back to me. It is not my job to create her perfect death. And even though an aspect of my life is dying (or transforming), it is not my death. I cannot control what her death will be like; it is in God's hands. At the same time, I realized that part of my desire was to give her a loving and heartfelt gift. So, I decided to create a ritual around giving up or letting go of the gift of the perfect death that I've been trying to give her and to acknowledge that I don't know, that none of us knows, what death is "supposed to" be.

As you go through this and the next exercise, you will identify the gift you hoped to give, symbolically wrap it up in a gift box, and offer it to God in a ceremony.

The Ritual Recipe

Part One: What Is the Perfect Death?

Journal about what you think is the perfect death. What is your ideal way to die? What are you hoping for the person you are care partnering with in terms of their death? Are there things you want

---

12. "The Eight Principles of Hospice Volunteering," presented during the Community Coalition Hospice volunteer training, Portland, OR, Jun 25, 2008.

to make happen for them before they die? Is there a particular quality to the way you hope their physical life will end?

_____

_____

_____

_____

_____

Part Two: The Logistics

Take some time to figure out the logistics for your ritual. Will it be just you? Will you invite others to support or to witness? Where would you like it to be? When would you like to do it? What time of day? What day of the week?

Who?

_____

_____

_____

_____

_____

Where?

_____

_____

_____

_____

_____

When?

_____

_____

_____

_____

_____

What prayers are significant to me and the person I am partnering with?

_____

_____

_____

_____

_____

Is there a particular song meaningful to either of us that I can use in this ritual?

_____

_____

_____

_____

_____

Part Three: Gather the ingredients:

The "ingredients" for this ritual are not the ingredients that will make your recipe "fail" if you don't use them. Substitutes and variations are encouraged. These are symbols to engage the senses (sight, sound, touch, smell, taste) that engage the heart and mind and are cues for you to remember that "church" is happening, that you are in sacred space. As you choose your ingredients, know that this ritual will be very personal and unique. Be creative.

The general ingredients needed are as follows:

- A flammable/composable object to represent your image of the perfect death. If you cannot find an object, simply write "the perfect death" on a piece of paper and put that in the box. You will know what it signifies, and God will, too.

- A box large enough to fit that object or paper.

- Wrapping paper and string/yarn from natural materials (flammable if you plan to burn it) to wrap the box/gift symbolizing your gratitude for this person.

- A source of fire to burn the gift or a shovel and a place to bury the gift.

- Choose a reading or two from a Bible or other sacred text that is meaningful to you and the person to whom you want to offer the perfect death.

- Select a song(s) and find a source for music (either prerecorded or have an instrument ready if you play, like a drum, rattle, or flute, or use your voice and sing).

- Bring an image of Jesus, Mary, a saint, or an ancestor that is meaningful to you as a symbol of their witness to this ritual.

- Sage, incense, or a candle (all optional) to help gather your awareness that this is a sacred space.

EXERCISE TWENTY-SEVEN | RITUAL— LETTING GO OF THE PERFECT DEATH

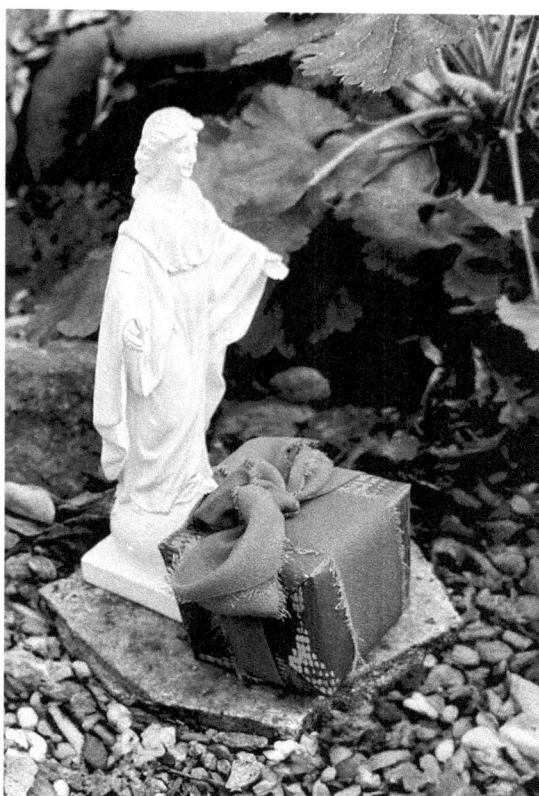

This image is from my own expression of this ritual for my stepmom, where I used a statue of Our Lady of the Smile to represent the loving witness of the divine.

The Ritual Enactment

As you begin this ritual, take the time to be clear on your purpose. Purpose, being focused on the "why" of what you are doing, is one of the critical components of a successful gathering or ritual.[13] Do this by bringing to mind and heart the gift you wish you could give this person and, when you are ready, acknowledging that it is a gift you cannot give. It is not yours to give. The serenity prayer might be helpful here:

"God, grant me the serenity to accept the things I cannot change; Courage to change the things I can; and Wisdom to know the difference."[14]

Take the object that symbolizes the perfect death you have wanted to give. Take that object and begin to place it in the box. As you do so, say to yourself or aloud what you wish you could give this person and how much you love and honor them. Pour your love and your desire to give to them into that box and then wrap it in wrapping paper that the PLwD would enjoy. This can be done ahead of time and on a different day than the ceremony if needed or if you would like to pray over the gift before offering it to God.

Now that you have your gift wrapped and ready to offer, prepare the area for your ritual. If you are going to burn your present, safely start a fire (and make sure you have water to put it out nearby). If you will bury it, ensure the area is clear and ready to receive your gift. It is helpful to dig the hole ahead of time. You can also do it during the releasing ritual. Then, gather the rest of your ingredients, including the present, and place them on the sacred ground of your ritual.

Feel free to modify the wording of the outline below to personalize it.

13. Parker, *Art of Gathering*, 1.

14. This prayer is credited to Dr. Reinhold Niebuhr of Union Theological Seminary. Wing, "Origin of the Serenity Prayer," 12.

Opening Prayer:

> *In the name of God, I ask all willing beings of God's love to be present with me (us) now. I invite Jesus, Mary, and Saint Joseph, the patron of good deaths. I call on my guardian angel(s) and on the guardian angel of [Name] and on our ancestors. Dear God, we gather today because I have taken on a burden that was not mine. [Name] has given me so much, and I am grateful. To repay them and honor you, oh God, I have wanted to create a perfect death for them. I have tried to manage every moment, every situation, to make it worthy of you, God, and to make it worthy of [Name].*
>
> *Dear God, I am tired, and in my weariness, I realize that this desire is not something I can do. Only you, God, know what this death is to look like. Only you, God, can make it holy. So, I invite you to take the weight of this burden as I can no longer carry it.*

Readings:

At this point, offer the prayer, poem, or Scripture reading(s) meaningful to you and your care partner. As you recite these readings, remember that as you speak their words, they become threads that join you with every living being that has ever read them, expanding the ritual beyond the borders of time.

Moment of Silence:

Take a moment of silence to sense the presence of God, the presence of love.

The Offering:

Now take the wrapped present and hold it near the flame (or over the hole you will place it in), and say a prayer of offering:

God, please take this gift, the gift of how I envision [Name]'s death. It was not mine to give, so I return it to you now. Forgive me for trying to take from you that which is yours to give. God, release me from this burden I have placed upon myself.

Song, Hymn, or Music:

As you place the present on the fire and watch it burn (or in the hole and cover the hole with dirt), play, sing, or perform the song/music you have prepared to honor this moment, the relationship you have with your care partner and the graces of God. As you do so, imagine all of the energy you have been holding around this pour into God's hands through the flame or through the earth.

Gratitude/Closing Prayer:

Once the music is completed and the present is released (fully burned or buried), say a prayer of gratitude:

Dear God, Thank you for the gift of [Name]. Thank you for hearing my cry for help. Thank you for being willing and caring hands into which I can place my burdens and my whole life. Thank you for the fire, the earth, and the angels you send to watch over us. Please help me live more attentively to your will and what you ask me to do. Continue to watch over [Name] and me as we continue this partnership of care together. Help us to love you more and grow closer to you each day. Amen.

Journal:

After cleaning up from the ritual and ensuring the fire is out, journal about your experience. What did it feel like? Did you notice any shifts in your awareness? In your body? Did you have a sense of God's presence? Describe what it was like.

Retreat Exercises

_____

_____

_____

_____

_____

EXERCISE TWENTY-EIGHT |
GRATITUDE MOMENT

When I started working at the day program, a colleague told me that if I thought I was getting things right about 50 percent of the time, I should be happy because that was a *really* good day. Mistakes happen in the world of care partnering, and it is easy to feel like you are not enough. As you do it day in and day out, those feelings of inadequacy can grow and compound. Gratitude can help shift this way of thinking.

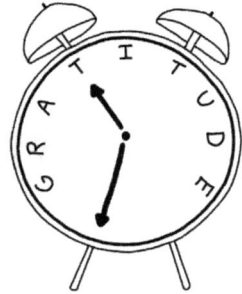

According to Brother Steindl-Rast, "When you are grateful, you act out of a sense of enough and not out of a sense of scarcity, and you are willing to share."[15] Acting out of a sense of enough, even when walking through the ever-changing landscape of the Valley of Dementia, would be completely revolutionary. And, if we had that sense of enoughness, how might that shift our generosity of care in relation to the PLwD? I invite you to try it out.

Take a few moments to ask the Holy Spirit to guide your attention to your role as a care partner and what aspects you like or bring you joy or satisfaction. Even if you don't particularly like the work itself, are there outcomes from the work you value or enjoy that make you feel good or connected to something bigger?

15. Dalai Lama XIV et al., *Book of Joy*, 246.

List three to five things (or more) you are grateful for about being a care partner. Then, take some time to offer a prayer of gratitude for these gifts and your awareness of them.

1.

2.

3.

4.

5.

EXERCISE TWENTY-NINE |
PRAYER—WORTHY OF GOD

God said, "I will put my laws in their minds, and I will write them upon their hearts" (Heb 8:10b NAB). God did not say, because they are so perfect, I will place my laws within them where they cannot be lost. When Jesus says, "You shall love the Lord, your God, with all your heart, with all your soul, and with all your mind" (Matt 22:37 NAB), God does not qualify these with conditions. One can have heart disease and still love with all of their heart. One can have dementia and still love with all of their mind. God's love is more vast than our understanding or ability. "You are the temple of God . . . the spirit of God dwells in you" (1 Cor 3:16 NAB).

> *Dear God, help me to know that you created me;*
> *that when I look in the mirror, I see a face of God,*
> *for I am made in your reflection.*
>
> *Please help me to see, when I look at my care partner,*
> *that I am gazing upon your face,*
> *for they, too, have been made in your likeness.*
>
> *Help me to release my assumptions about you and PLwD*
> *so that I might enter into a sacramental experience of the*
> *world,*
> *where every creature glorifies God,*
> *by offering its unique expression of God's grace and love.*
>
> *Help me to trust that you placed inside each of us*
> *what we need to follow Your law*
> *and that even when we are depleted,*
> *declining, impulsive, or making mistakes,*

what we have to offer you and each other is enough
because your decree, that which you have written inside
our very being,
and not our mistakes or imperfections will prevail
(Prov 19:21).

I offer you my every weakness,
for your power to be made perfect there (2 Cor 12:9).

Help me love you with everything I am
and guide my actions so that they each
become prayers and celebrations
of your compassion and your mercy.

Create for us, in this Valley of Dementia,
a safe and expansive place where we might
journey together in the fullness of Your love;

May we know that we are your beloved,
and so we are each other's beloved,
and may that give us the strength to take the next step.

In your name we pray.
Amen.

EXERCISE THIRTY | RITUAL—A
CELEBRATION OF GRATITUDE

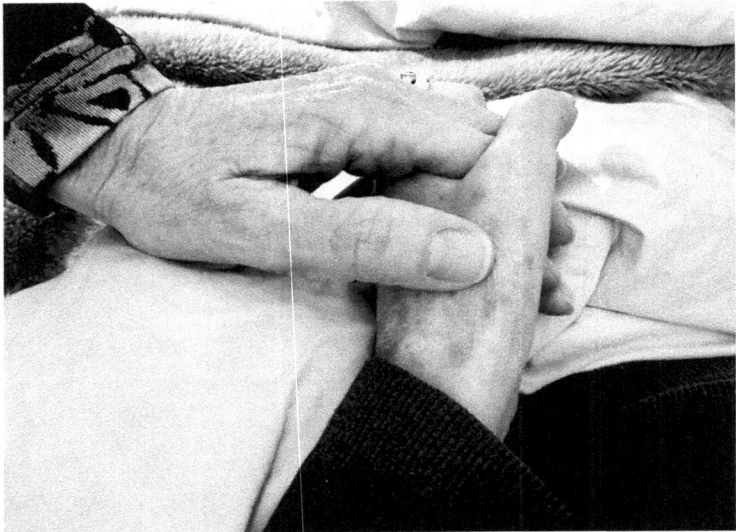

This exercise honors your completion of this retreat and your commitment to yourself, God, and PLwD. Whether or not you took time to engage in this spiritual retreat, you are not the same person as when you began care partnering in the Valley of Dementia. Life's journeys change us. Your choice to engage more deeply with God through this retreat has also changed you and helped to form your future. Hopefully, you have begun to see that everything you do as a care partner is a form of prayer; it is faith in action. As God invites PLwD closer each day, we also are invited closer to God each day, often through the PLwD. Both are acts of God's creation, through you letting go of the past and God making something new (Isa 43:18–19).

PLwD might not be aware of everything we do in our care partnering journey. That does not negate the value of what we are doing. Others might see us as wasting our time at the bedside of someone who is dying or who can no longer communicate or comprehend. Yet, we embody Christ through our service to someone God deeply loves.[16] In our care for PLwD, we are offering God's love. We are being God's church that does not abandon those in need. In this way, the PLwD offers us our ministerial work in the world. They provide us with the ability to act in the image of God. They allow us to say, over and over again, "yes" to God.

I invite you to close your retreat with a series of gratitudes. We learned earlier that secrets are detrimental to your health, so don't keep your gratitude a secret. Even if you journal it, that is enough. Or, share your appreciation in some form of communal prayer, with thank you notes, or in conversation.

First, thank the PLwD for who they have been for you throughout life and through the Valley of Dementia. The dementia that you both are experiencing is changing you both, giving you opportunities to grow closer to God. Second, thank your "sticky note friends" or anyone else who supported you, whether or not you reached out to them during this retreat. They, like God, have been present in your life and walked with you through this Valley of Dementia.

And remember, nothing can separate you and your care partner from the love of God (Rom 8:38–39), not dementia, not a bad day, not a care partnering mistake, not even the lack of a body. And death is not a failure. For many of us, getting closer to God has been our goal since the day we were born. During this retreat, you and the person you care partner have grown closer to God, each in your own way. May God's peace and grace be with you as you continue your life's journey, growing ever closer to God.

---

16. Saunders, *Dementia: Pastoral Theology*, 20.

IN CLOSING

A hospice chaplain once recommended that as we say goodbye to our loved ones, we tell them five things: "Thank you," "I'm sorry," "I forgive you," "I love you," and "goodbye." So, I would like to thank you for your commitment to this work, the people in your life, the sacredness of life and death, love, and God. Thank you for being willing to show up in all your messiness, listen to your heart and the heart of God, continue the journey, and not give up. Thank you for allowing me to share some of my life with you. Thank you for indulging in my love of spiritual and prayerful experimentation, which I believe is how we each learn our particular love language with the Divine. I am sorry if my words were unclear, inaccurate, or if I made you feel pressured to be something you are not. I am a human being, an imperfect work in progress. I forgive you for those days when you felt you "missed the mark." I love you just as you are, a face of God, a messy, spectacular, wonderful part of the unity of all things.

And, as this retreat comes to a close, I say goodbye for now and offer you this prayer, one of my stepmom's favorites, from the Night Prayer in *A New Zealand Prayer Book—He Karakia Mihinare o Aotearoa*.

> Lord,
> It is night.
>
> The night is for stillness.
> Let us be still in the presence of God.
>
> It is night after a long day.
> What has been done has been done;

what has not been done has not been done;
let it be.

The night is dark.
Let our fears of the darkness of the world and of our own
lives rest in you.

The night is quiet.
Let the quietness of your peace enfold us,
all dear to us,
and all who have no peace.

The night heralds the dawn.
Let us look expectantly to a new day,
new joys,
new possibilities.

In your name we pray.
Amen.

> *"Be steadfast and persevering, my beloved sisters and brothers, fully engaged in the work of Jesus. You know that your toil is not in vain when it is done in Christ."—1 Corinthians 15:58 TIB*

8

Additional Resources

ONLINE RECORDINGS OF EXERCISES MARKED WITH AN ASTERISK (*)

RECORDINGS OF SOME OF this retreat's exercises are available using this QR code or can be found at:

https:\\www.youtube.com/@ValleyofDementiaRetreat

IGNATIAN SPIRITUALITY

Though I have not spent time in this retreat explaining the structure and methodology of Ignatian spirituality, the work is heavily influenced by Ignatius' teachings on deepening one's personal relationship with the divine through prayer and scriptural engagement. For more information on Ignatian spirituality and the spiritual exercises, here are just a few resources available:

- *Draw Me into Your Friendship: The Spiritual Exercises* by David L. Fleming, S.J. This book presents the original translation of St. Ignatius' Spiritual Exercises side by side with more contemporary language that can help you understand and apply the text to your life.

- *The Ignatian Adventure: Experiencing the Spiritual Exercises of Saint Ignatius in Daily Life* by Kevin O'Brien. This book is a self-directed version of the spiritual exercises of St. Ignatius.

- The Ignatian Spirituality Institute provides general information on Ignatian Spirituality on their website. https://ignatianinstitute.org/

- Check with your local church or retreat centers, which might offer a version of the spiritual exercises if you decide that might benefit you.

- Boston College's Institute for Advanced Jesuit Studies offers a twelve-week Ignatian retreat each summer that you can do on your own or in conjunction with a faith-sharing group. https://www.bc.edu/content/bc-web/centers/iajs/programs/retreat.html

- "Pray as You Go" is a website and a free app that guides you through short daily prayer experiences based on Ignatian Spirituality. https://pray-as-you-go.org/

DEMENTIA CARE

Teepa Snow is a leading expert on Dementia Care, using what she calls *A Positive Approach to Dementia Care*.[1]

- Her book *Understanding the Changing Brain* offers an understanding of how the brain functions, how it loses function

1. Snow, *Understanding the Changing Brain*.

as it dies, and how care partners can adapt their approach to share a better quality of life.

- Her website, www.teepasnow.com, offers formal training opportunities (both free and for a fee), general information on care advice, and an explanation of her trademarked GEMS® Brain Change Model that can help you recognize the characteristics of where a PLwD's cognitive abilities are and how care partners can use that information to interact more effectively.

- Many of her instructional videos are available on YouTube. https://www.youtube.com/@teepasnowvideos/

TRAUMA CARE

There are a lot of books, workbooks, and other materials on trauma and trauma recovery that you can find easily with a quick internet search. However, if trauma is something that is coming up for you very acutely amid your care partnering journey, you might consider finding a therapist who can accompany you. Trauma is complicated, and the exhaustive efforts of care partnering can trigger it or complicate it even more.

Many therapists can meet via Zoom or other telehealth modalities if you cannot leave the house easily. If you are employed, check to see if you have an Employee Assistance Program. Many of these offer free counseling services. If you are not, check with your health care provider to see if counseling is covered under your health insurance or check with your local church office or other community support organizations. Though I don't know the details of your specific community recourses, I do know that there are people out there who care and want to help. If you find yourself in crisis, some emergency resources include the following:

- Crisis Text Line (for any crisis): 741741
- Substance Abuse and Mental Health Line: 1 (800) 662–4357 or text 435–748

- Suicide Prevention Lifeline: 1 (800) 273-TALK(8255)
- Veterans Crisis Line 1 (800) 273–8255 and press 1

OTHER SUPPORT GROUPS/SERVICES, INCLUDING HOSPICE

- The Alzheimer's Association website has all sorts of information about Alzheimer's, including classes and listings of local or virtual support groups. https://www.alz.org/help-support.

- Check with your local or state government for Area Agencies on Aging. They often offer advice and resources such as classes and support groups and can refer you to other agencies and people for additional help if needed.

- Look to see if your area has an Adult Day Program. These are places where the PLwD can go for the day and participate in all sorts of activities, including exercise, art, games, meals, and social engagement, while getting personalized assistance ensuring their safety and comfort. These organizations also often offer support groups for care partners and brain fitness programs for persons living with dementia.

- Hospice and palliative care are resources that can support you on your journey and focus on comfort care, symptom management, and improving quality of life. Hospice services require a doctor's declaration that a person is terminally ill and is expected to live six months or less. There are both private and not-for-profit hospice organizations. You have the right to choose the hospice organization that is right for you. It is okay to interview agencies before signing up for hospice to see if they have the kind of care team you seek. Hospice organizations provide a team that includes a social worker, chaplain, nurse, home health aide, and sometimes a trained volunteer to support you and your partner in the latter stages of this journey. The hospice team can help with everything from bathing to medication management to funeral planning and often offers support groups for care partners, including anticipatory grief groups and bereavement services. Depending on the agency, volunteer services can include respite, spiritual care, companionship, and comfort therapies such as art therapy, reiki or touch therapy, and sound therapy. You have the right to switch agencies if they do not meet your needs, and you have the right to take the PLwD off of hospice services.

- Another resource available to you as you enter the latter stages of the dementia journey is the Threshold Choir. Threshold Choir is an international organization of volunteers who bring comfort and a caring presence singing for those at the thresholds of life. More information, including video samples and locations of chapters, can be found on their website: https://thresholdchoir.org/.

About the Author

THERESE FISHER BRINGS A wealth of compassion and an intimate understanding of the challenges and joys of dementia care into this retreat. With more than fifteen years of expertise in hospice care and a background in sound healing, spiritual direction, reiki, and singing with the Threshold Choir and the Mount Calvary Baptist Church mass choir (https://mcbcfs.org), her work reflects her unwavering commitment to providing companionship, respite, and assistance to those in need.

As a dedicated member of the care team of her stepmother, who has lived with Alzheimer's disease for more than a decade, and in her role as a person-centered care specialist in an Adult Day Health Care facility, Therese's personal and professional experiences have fostered profound empathy that resonates in her work. Holding a master's degree in theological studies from the Jesuit School of Theology of Santa Clara University, her academic pursuits have further enriched her capacity to offer holistic guidance to care partners. Her self-paced spiritual retreat is a testament to her love of God, her Jesuit education, and her commitment to helping others discover peace, understanding, and connection within the complexities of life and through dementia care. https://theresefisher.com

Bibliography

Acharya, Sourya, and Samarth Shukla. "Mirror Neurons: Enigma of the Metaphysical Modular Brain." *Journal of Natural Science, Biology, and Medicine* 3.2 (2012) 118–24. https://www.ncbi.nlm.nih.gov/pmc/articles/PMC3510904/.

"Adult Day Health." Providence Community Health Foundation Napa Valley, n.d. https://foundation.providence.org/ca/napa/our-priorities/adult-day-health.

Alzheimer's Association. *Alzheimer's Disease Facts and Figures.* Chicago, IL: Alzheimer's Association, 2007.

The Anglican Church in Aotearoa, New Zealand, and Polynesia. *A New Zealand Prayer Book—He Karakia Mihinare o Aotearoa.* San Francisco: HarperOne, 1997.

Baldovin, John F. *Bread of Life, Cup of Salvation: Understanding the Mass.* Lanham, MD: Rowan & Littlefield, 2003.

Blackaby, Henry, et al. *Experiencing God: Knowing and Doing the Will of God.* Brentwood, TN: Lifeway, 2022.

Bonhoeffer, Dietrich, and Walter Brueggemann. *Psalms: The Prayer Book of the Bible.* Old Saybrook, CT: Christian Audio, 2022.

Brodaty, Henry, and Marika Donkin. "Family Caregivers of People with Dementia." *Dialogues in Clinical Neuroscience* 11.2 (June 2009) 217–28. https://doi.org/10.31887/DCNS.2009.11.2/hbrodaty.

Brueggemann, Walter. *From Whom No Secrets Are Hid: Introducing the Psalms.* 1st ed. Louisville: Westminster John Knox, 2014.

Chittister, Joan. *The Monastic Heart: 50 Simple Practices for a Contemplative and Fulfilling Life.* New York: Convergent, 2021.

Dalai Lama XIV, et al. *The Book of Joy: Lasting Happiness in a Changing World.* New York: Avery, 2016.

Damjanovic, Amanda K., et al. "Accelerated Telomere Erosion is Associated with a Declining Immune Function of Caregivers of Alzheimer's Disease Patients." *Journal of Immunology* 179.6 (September 15, 2007) 4249–54. https://doi.org/10.4049/jimmunol.179.6.4249.

Bibliography

Davis, Robert, and Betty Davis. *My Journey into Alzheimer's Disease.* 1st ed. Wheaton, IL: Tyndale, 1989.

Day, Jennifer R., and Ruth A. Anderson. "Compassion Fatigue: An Application of the Concept to Informal Caregivers of Family Members with Dementia." *Nursing Research and Practice* 2011 (2011). https://doi.org/10.1155/2011/408024.

"Dementia." World Health Organization, Mar 15, 2023. https://www.who.int/news-room/fact-sheets/detail/dementia.

Driver, Tom F. *Liberating Rites: Understanding the Transformative Power of Ritual.* N.p.: BookSurge, 2006.

Evangelical Presbyterian Church. *Westminster Confession of Faith.* 15th ed. Orlando: Evangelical Presbyterian Church, 2017.

Feurich, Valerie. "Teepa Snow's 10 Steps to De-escalating a Dementia Care Crisis: Strategies for Calming a Person in Acute Distress." Positive Approach to Care, Jul 8, 2021. https://teepasnow.com/blog/teepa-snows-10-steps-to-de-escalating-a-dementia-care-crisis/.

Flemming, David L. *Draw Me Into Your Friendship: A Literal Translation and a Contemporary Reading of The Spiritual Exercises.* 1st ed. St. Louis: Institute of Jesuit Sources, 1996.

Fleurdujon, Devin. "Rite of Passage in the Loss of One of Our Greatest Common Rituals: Eating!" Flipgrid, Apr 2023. https://flip.com/663c0498.

Francis. *Amoris Laetitia.* Vatican City: Liberia Editrice Vaticana, 2016.

———. "*Evangelii Gaudium*": *Apostolic Exhortation on the Proclamation of the Gospel in Today's World.*" The Holy See, Nov 24, 2013. https://www.vatican.va/content/francesco/en/apost_exhortations/documents/papa-francesco_esortazione-ap_20131124_evangelii-gaudium.html.

Grimes, Ronald L. *Deeply into the Bone: Re-inventing Rites of Passage.* Berkeley, CA: University of California Press, 2000.

Gundar-Goshen, Ayelet. "Trauma: A Conversation with Israeli Author and Psychologist Ayelet Gundar-Goshen." Vimeo, Oct 23, 2023. https://vimeo.com/881872788.

Hauerwas, Stanley. *God, Medicine, and Suffering.* Grand Rapids: Eerdmans, 1994.

———. "Must a Patient Be a Person to Be a Patient?" *Journal of Religion, Disability and Health* 8.3–4 (Feb 24, 2005) 113–19. https://doi.org/10.1300/J095v08n03_13.

Kessler, David. *Finding Meaning: The Sixth Stage of Grief.* New York: Scribner, 2019.

Kiecolt-Glaser, J. K., et al. "Spousal Caregivers of Dementia Victims: Longitudinal Changes in Immunity and Health." *Psychosomatic Medicine* 53.4 (July 1991) 345–62. https://doi.org/10.1097/00006842–199107000-00001.

Lane, Belden C. *Ravished by Beauty: The Surprising Legacy of Reformed Spirituality.* New York: Oxford University Press, 2011.

Bibliography

"The Later Stage of Dementia." Alzheimer's Society, Jun 18, 2021. https://www.alzheimers.org.uk/about-dementia/symptoms-and-diagnosis/how-dementia-progresses/later-stages-dementia.

Liebert, Elizabeth, and Annemarie Paulin-Campbell. *The Spiritual Exercises Reclaimed, 2nd Edition: Uncovering Liberating Possibilities for Women.* New York: Paulist, 2022.

Martin, Calvin Luther. *The Way of the Human Being.* New Haven, CT: Yale University Press, 1999.

Maté, Gabor, and Daniel Maté. *The Myth of Normal: Trauma, Illness and Healing in a Toxic Culture.* New York: Avery, 2022. Kindle ed.

Moltmann, Jürgen. *The Crucified God.* Minneapolis: Fortress, 2015.

Parker, Priya. *The Art of Gathering: How We Meet and Why It Matters.* New York: Riverhead, 2018.

Paul VI. "Constitution on the Sacred Liturgy Sacrosanctum Concilium." The Holy See, Dec 4, 1963. https://www.vatican.va/archive/hist_councils/ii_vatican_council/documents/vat-ii_const_19631204_sacrosanctum-concilium_en.html.

Pennebaker, James W., and Joshua M. Smyth. *Opening Up by Writing It Down: How Expressive Writing Improves Health and Eases Emotional Pain.* New York: Guilford, 2016. Kindle ed.

Pontifical Biblical Commission. "What Is Man? An Itinerary of Biblical Anthropology." The Holy See, 2019. https://www.vatican.va/roman_curia/congregations/cfaith/pcb_documents/rc_con_cfaith_doc_20190930_cosa-e-luomo_it.html.

Rilke, Rainer Maria. *Letters to a Young Poet.* Translated by Joan Burnham. Novato, CA: New World Library, 2000.

Sanders, Sara. "Is the Glass Half Empty or Half Full? Reflections on Strain and Gain in Caregivers of Individuals with Alzheimer's Disease." *Social Work in Health Care* 40.3 (January 2005) 57–73. https://doi.org/10.1300/J010v40n03_04.

Saunders, James. *Dementia: Pastoral Theology and Pastoral Care.* Grove Pastoral Series P89. Cambridge: Grove, 2002.

Shapiro, Alison Bonds. "Mirroring Care." *Psychology Today,* Sep 17, 2010. https://www.psychologytoday.com/us/blog/healing-possibility/201009/mirroring-care.

Shin, Ji Hye, and Ji Hyun Kim. "Family Caregivers of People with Dementia Associate with Poor Health-Related Quality of Life: A Nationwide Population-Based Study." *International Journal of Environmental Research and Public Health* 19.23 (December 2022). https://doi.org/10.3390%2Fijerph192316252.

Snow, Teepa. "Innovative Approaches to Dementia Care with Teepa Snow." Training event at Crosswalk Community Church, Napa, CA, May 12, 2022.

———. *Understanding the Changing Brain: A Positive Approach to Dementia Care.* Efland, NC: Positive Approach, 2021.

Bibliography

———. "What Are The GEMS®?" Positive Approach to Care, n.d. https://teepasnow.com/about-dementia/#pacskills.

Swinton, John. *Dementia: Living in the Memories of God.* Grand Rapids: Eerdmans, 2012.

"Virtual Dementia Tour." Second Wind Dreams, n.d. https://www.secondwind.org/virtual-dementia-tourreg.html.

Wing, Nell. "Origin of the Serenity Prayer: A Historical Paper." Alcoholics Anonymous, Jul 30, 2009. https://www.aa.org/sites/default/files/literature/assets/smf-129_en.pdf.

www.ingramcontent.com/pod-product-compliance
Lightning Source LLC
Chambersburg PA
CBHW070250290326
41930CB00041B/2431

9798385215874